Introduction to Resting State fMRI
Functional Connectivity

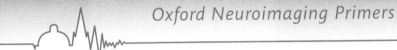

*Oxford Neuroimaging Primers*

OXFORD NEUROIMAGING PRIMERS

# Introduction to
# Resting State fMRI
# Functional Connectivity

JANINE BIJSTERBOSCH

STEPHEN SMITH

CHRISTIAN BECKMANN

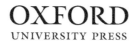

OXFORD

UNIVERSITY PRESS

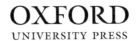

# OXFORD
## UNIVERSITY PRESS

Great Clarendon Street, Oxford, OX2 6DP,
United Kingdom

Oxford University Press is a department of the University of Oxford.
It furthers the University's objective of excellence in research, scholarship,
and education by publishing worldwide. Oxford is a registered trade mark of
Oxford University Press in the UK and in certain other countries

First Edition published in 2017

Impression: 9

Published in the United States of America by Oxford University Press
198 Madison Avenue, New York, NY 10016, United States of America

British Library Cataloguing in Publication Data
Data available

Library of Congress Control Number: 2017938214

ISBN 978-0-19-880822-0

Printed in Great Britain by
Ashford Colour Press Ltd, Gosport, Hampshire

# Preface to the Series

The Oxford Neuroimaging Primers are aimed to be readily accessible texts for new researchers or advanced undergraduates from the biological, medical or physical sciences. They are intended to provide a broad understanding of the ways in which neuroimaging data can be analyzed and interpreted. All primers in this series have been written so that they can be read as stand-alone books, although they have also been edited so that they "work together," and readers can read multiple primers in the series to build up a bigger picture of neuroimaging and be equipped to use multiple neuroimaging methods.

Understanding the principles of the analysis of neuroimaging data is crucial for all researchers in this field, not only because data analysis is a necessary part of any neuroimaging study, but also because it is required in order to understand how to plan, execute, and interpret experiments. Although MR operators, radiologists, and technicians are often available to help with data collection, running the scanner and choosing good sequences and settings, when it comes to analysis, researchers are often on their own. Therefore the Oxford Neuroimaging Primers seek to provide the necessary understanding in how to do analysis at the same time trying to show how this knowledge relates to being able to perform good acquisitions, design good experiments and correctly interpret the results.

The series has been produced by individuals (both authors and editors) who have developed neuroimaging analysis techniques, used these methods on real data, packaged them as software tools for others to use, taught courses on these methods and supported people around the world who use the software they have produced. We hope that this means everyone involved has both the experience to instruct, but also the empathy to support the reader. It has been our aim for these primers to not only lay out the core principles that apply in any given area of neuroimaging, but also to help the reader avoid common pitfalls and mistakes (many of which the authors themselves probably made first). We also hope that the series is also a good introduction to those with a more technical background, even if they have to forgo some of the mathematical details found in other more technical works. We make no pretence that these primers are the final word in any given area, and the field of neuroimaging continues to develop and improve, but the fundamentals are likely to remain the same for many years to come. Certainly some of the advice you will find in the primers will never fail you, such as *always look at your data*.

Our intention with the series was always to support it with practical examples, so that the reader can learn from working with data directly and will be equipped to use the knowledge they gained in their own studies and on their own data. These examples, including datasets and instructions, can be found on the associated website (www.neuroimagingprimers.org) and directions to specific examples are placed throughout each primer. As the authors are also the developers of various software tools within the FMRIB Software Library (FSL), the examples in the primers mainly use tools from FSL. However, we intend these primers to be as general as possible and present material that is relevant for all readers, regardless of the software they use in practice. Such readers can still use the example data available through the primer website with any of the major neuroimaging analysis toolboxes. We encourage all readers to interact with these examples, as we strongly believe that a lot of the key learning is done when you actually use these tools in practice.

Mark Jenkinson
Michael Chappell
Oxford, January 2017

# Preface

Welcome to this primer on an *Introduction to Resting State fMRI Functional Connectivity*, which is part of a series of Oxford NeuroImaging Primers. This primer is aimed at people who are new to the field of resting state fMRI and functional connectivity. For many people who fit into this category, the large variety of approaches to functional connectivity analysis is highly confusing. This primer aims to provide an overview of the concepts and analysis decisions that need to be made at every step of the analysis pipeline for resting state fMRI data, including issues of data acquisition and the interpretation of findings. Our intention was to introduce a wide range of analysis approaches without relying on any particular experience or prerequisite knowledge, making this primer accessible to people from a broad range of different backgrounds. This primer does assume some general background knowledge on functional magnetic resonance imaging (fMRI), and if you are entirely new to fMRI you may benefit from reading the introductory primer for this series first.

This primer contains several different types of boxes in the text that are aimed to help you navigate the material or find out more information for yourself. To get the most out of this primer, you might find the descriptions of each type of box below helpful.

**Example box** These boxes direct you to the Oxford NeuroImaging Primers website: www.neuroimagingprimers.org, where you will find examples that allow you to directly interact with data and perform practical exercises to apply the theory described in this primer. These examples are intended to be a useful way to prepare you for applying these methods to your own data, but you do not need to carry out these examples as you read through the primer. The examples are placed at the relevant places in the text so that you know when you can get a more hands-on approach to the information being presented.

> **Example box: Single subject**
>
> To get a better feel for the types
> a look at the ICA components t
> the primer website you will find

**Box** These boxes contain more technical or advanced descriptions of some topics covered in this primer or information on related topics or methods. None of the material in the rest of the primer assumes that you have read these boxes, and they are not essential for understanding and applying any of the methods. If you are new to the field and are reading this primer for the first time, you may therefore prefer to skip the material in these boxes and come back to them later.

> **Box 1.1 Neuronal activity**
>
> Inputs are transferred from one n
> via the release of chemicals calle
> cleft that exists between axon ter

**General statistics box:** Multi

This box contains a brief introduc
ysis, because this is the approach
book, namely:

**General statistics box** This primer includes a couple of longer boxes that describe some general statistics material that is needed to prepare you for running your own analyses (i.e., these boxes should not be skipped). These boxes contain material that is relevant to many different topics covered in different chapters in this primer, and it is therefore written in relatively general terms.

## SUMMARY

■ The BOLD signal measured in activity (which can be measur

■ Spontaneous BOLD fluctuati across brain regions in a way

**Summary** Each chapter contains a box of summary points towards the end, which provide a very brief overview, emphasizing the most important topics discussed in each chapter. You may like to use these to check that you have understood the key points in each chapter.

## FURTHER READING

■ Biswal, B., Yetkin, F.Z., Haugh the motor cortex of resting *in Medicine: Official Journal c Magnetic Resonance in Medi*

**Further reading** Each chapter ends with a list of suggestions for further reading, including both articles and books. A brief summary of the contents of each suggestion is included, so that you can choose which references are most relevant to you. None of the material in this primer assumes that you have read any of the further reading material. Rather, these lists suggest a starting point for diving deeper into the existing literature. These boxes are not intended to provide a full review of the relevant literature; should you go further into the field you will find a wealth of other sources that are helpful or important for the specific research you are doing.

Resting state functional connectivity is a research field that is still at a relatively early stage, that is evolving rapidly, and will most likely continue to do so over the coming years. Therefore, the aim of this primer is to provide a comprehensive and introductory overview of the most commonly used approaches. We hope that this will provide good preparation for delving into the vast literature on resting state fMRI.

Janine Bijsterbosch
Stephen Smith
Christian Beckmann

# Acknowledgments

Many people have contributed to the writing of this primer. In particular, I am grateful to the editors for giving me the opportunity to write this primer, and specifically to Mark Jenkinson for his continued support and enthusiasm during the writing process. I am also grateful to my coauthors, Christian and Steve, for their insightful comments and the interesting discussions that developed while writing this primer. Furthermore, I would like to thank Zobair Arya, Jon Campbell, Michael Chappell, Falk Eippert, Stefania Evangelisti, Olivia Faull, Ludovica Griffanti, Sam Harrison, Saad Jbabdi, Mark Jenkinson, Fred Lenz, Paul McCarthy, Thomas Nichols, Michael Sanders, Charlotte Stagg, and Anderson Winkler for proofreading and commenting on earlier versions of this primer. I would also like to thank Paul McCarthy for his help with creating the cover image. Finally, I would like to thank my husband, Maarten Vooijs, for proofreading, and for his continual encouragement, support, and patience.

Janine Bijsterbosch

# Contents

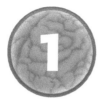

# Introduction

The human brain represents about 2% of our overall body weight, yet it is thought to consume approximately 20% of the total amount of energy produced by our body, even when it is not performing any particular cognitive task. This fact has intrigued researchers for decades. What does the brain do when we are apparently not doing anything? How does this intrinsic activity relate to cognition, personality, disease, and consciousness? Interest in *intrinsic activity* (as opposed to extrinsic activity, which occurs in response to external stimuli) has steadily increased over the years, and with advances in functional magnetic resonance imaging (fMRI), studying the brain's activity level during rest using so called "resting state fMRI," has bloomed into a research field in its own right.

Aimed at researchers that are new to the field of resting state fMRI, this book introduces the major concepts and analysis approaches. In the interest of brevity, this primer does not cover all the technical details, or every possible approach. Rather, an overview is presented, and it is hoped that this will provide good preparation for delving into the vast literature on resting state fMRI. Please note that this book specifically does not explain functional MRI itself more generally, and people who are new to fMRI in general may find it helpful to read the primer *Introduction to Neuroimaging Analysis* that is also part of this series.

## 1.1 From neural activity to functional connectivity

On a general level, there are two overarching concepts in the field of neuroimaging that can inform us about how the brain works. The first of these is *localization*, which aims to assign functions to specific regions of the brain. Many researchers use carefully designed behavioral tasks that subjects perform in the MRI scanner in order to localize functionally specialized regions of the brain that activate in response to a specific aspect of behavior. Tasks typically include multiple different conditions (including baseline periods), and task-induced activation is measured and localized by comparing the blood oxygen level dependent (BOLD) signal between different conditions. The second general concept is to investigate *connectivity*, or the way in which brain regions communicate with one another and information is passed from one brain area to the next. In order to investigate connectivity, we measure the similarity of the BOLD signals from different brain regions, because if the signals are similar, this is likely to mean that the regions are passing on information from one region to the other (i.e., there is connectivity). In order to study connectivity, we often look at spontaneous fluctuations in the signal, when there are no specific cognitive demands for the subject (so-called resting state scans). Using spontaneous fluctuations allows us to investigate similarity between regions when it is not biased by any specific task. As such, resting state fMRI has emerged as a valuable way to study brain connectivity. For the purpose of this book, "rest" or "resting state" are defined as being awake, but not performing any specific task (unless otherwise stated).

The previous paragraph describes the ideas and concepts that people refer to when they talk about *localization* and *connectivity*. It is useful to understand how these concepts relate to physiological processes in the brain both at the neuronal level and at the macroscopic level that we measure in fMRI (Figure 1.1). At the microscopic level, a neuron consists of a cell body (soma) that receives input through dendrites and passes action potentials through axonal tracts to other cells. These microscopic processes in turn result in a localized increase in blood flow that far exceeds the oxygen demands of the neural activity, leading to a local increase in blood oxygenation level (Figure 1.1). It is crucial to appreciate that BOLD fMRI measures this increase in blood oxygenation, which is a secondary and indirect measure of neuronal activity. The hemodynamic response to neural activity which is measured in fMRI (i.e., blood oxygenation levels) is a relatively slow process that only reaches its peak approximately 5–6 seconds after the start of the neural activity. Using concurrent fMRI and electrophysiological recording, previous research has shown a strong link between spontaneous fluctuations in resting state

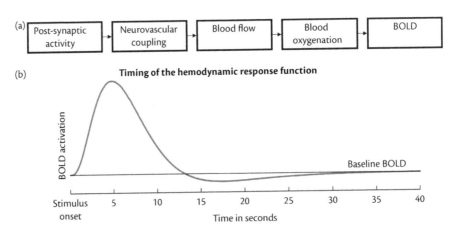

**Figure 1.1:** The BOLD signal is an indirect measure of neuronal activity that is mediated by a slow increase in local oxygenated blood flow that takes several seconds to peak. (a) Several complex biological processes such as neurovascular coupling take place, which together result in the localized increases in blood oxygenation that are measured in BOLD fMRI. (b) The standard form of the hemodynamic response function is shown. From stimulus onset, the BOLD signal takes approximately 5 seconds to reach its maximum.

BOLD data and slow fluctuations in the local field potential (LFP). Therefore, the BOLD signal is thought to primarily reflect the excitatory inputs to the neural population (synchronized post-synaptic activity). The relationship between resting state functional connectivity and local neurophysiology is discussed in more detail in Chapter 6.

---

**Box 1.1: Neuronal activity and local field potential**

Inputs are transferred from one neuron's axon terminal to the dendrites of another neuron via the release of chemicals called neurotransmitters (such as glutamate) into the synaptic cleft that exists between axon terminals and dendrites. Activity in a population of neurons can therefore be measured by either looking at the firing rate (the overall pattern of spikes or action potentials), or by measuring the LFP, which reflects a summation of the synchronized post-synaptic activity. The relationship between the firing rate and the LFP is complex because an increase in post-synaptic activity may affect different groups of neurons in different ways and does therefore not simply result in an increase in population firing rate. The physiological basis of BOLD is discussed in more detail in Chapter 6.

---

Functional connectivity is typically defined as: "the observed temporal correlation (or other statistical dependencies) between two electro- or neurophysiological measurements from different parts of the brain." For resting state fMRI this definition means that functional connectivity can inform us about the relationship between BOLD signals obtained from two separate regions of the brain. The underlying assumption is that if two regions show similarities in their BOLD signals over time, they are functionally connected.

Many different methods exist to look at such similarities, and several are covered in more detail in this book. The simplest way to investigate similarity between two signals is by looking at their timeseries *correlation* using Pearson's correlation coefficient. Correlation ranges from −1 (perfect negative correlation) to +1 (perfect positive correlation), where 0 indicates no relationship on average between two signals. In 1995, Biswal and colleagues compared task activation maps during finger tapping with a map of correlation coefficients of BOLD data obtained during a scan when the subject was resting. The resting state correlation map was created by taking all voxels that were activated by the motor task and using only the resting state data to calculate the correlation of each voxel in the brain with those "activated" voxels. The task activation map and resulting resting state correlation map showed strong spatial similarities. This work is now often cited as the first study to show that intrinsic fluctuations measured in the brain at rest by functional MRI hold information about the inherent functional organization of the human brain. The spatial structure of functionally connected regions, which is consistently and reliably found in resting state fMRI data, forms the foundation for resting state fMRI research. Therefore, while functional connectivity is defined in terms of temporal similarity between signals, the spatial patterns that emerge when looking at connectivity are often of primary interest in functional connectivity research.

It is important to distinguish functional connectivity from other types of connectivity. First, while functional connectivity describes the relationship between two regions, it is not typically used to describe directionality (also called causality, which refers to a situation where the signal from one region is responsible for driving the signal in a second region). This type of directed connectivity is described by *effective connectivity*. Directionality and causality are challenging topics to study in BOLD fMRI data, and this is discussed further in Chapter 6. Secondly, it is tempting to interpret functional connectivity as a direct physical connection (e.g., an axonal white matter tract) between two brain regions. However, this type of *anatomical connectivity* cannot be inferred from functional connectivity results alone. These different types of connectivity will be discussed in more detail in Chapter 6, but the majority of this book will focus on functional connectivity estimated from BOLD fMRI recordings.

Many different methodological approaches to studying functional connectivity are available and several of these will be discussed in more detail in Chapters 4 and 5. While some of these analysis approaches may appear very different from one another at first glance, it is important to realize that all methods discussed in this work are based on the definition of functional connectivity described above. Therefore, the field of resting state functional connectivity revolves around detecting similarities among distinct regions of the brain. Specifically, in the case of functional connectivity MRI, we detect similarities between the BOLD signal measured in different parts of the brain.

## 1.2   What is a resting state network (RSN)?

A group or system of interconnected people or things is often called a network. Think, for example, about your social media network or a computer network. Given the definition of functional connectivity described above, a *resting state network* is simply a set of brain regions that show similarities in their BOLD timeseries obtained during rest. At present, we do not have a complete understanding of the network structure of the resting brain. Nonetheless, several networks can be reproducibly found using a variety of analysis approaches.

Different resting state networks have been identified and "named" mostly on the basis of the spatial similarity between the resting state networks and activation patterns seen in task fMRI experiments. This naming convention is most accurate for areas associated with sensory processing, where it has been established that a correspondence exists between areas that can be mapped in response to sensory stimulation and areas that have strong resting state BOLD similarities. Other parts of the brain, for example within multimodal association cortex, are more ambiguously related to task experiments.

Perhaps the best-known resting state network of all is the *Default Mode Network* (DMN; Figure 1.2). The DMN contains regions in the brain that consistently show decreases in activity when the brain is performing any type of task compared with rest (*deactivations*), as shown by early task-based imaging studies using both fMRI and positron emission tomography (PET). Key regions of the DMN are the posterior cingulate cortex, precuneus, medial prefrontal cortex, inferior parietal lobule, and lateral temporal cortex.

The *dorsal attention network* (DAN; also called the task-positive network; Figure 1.2) is another commonly described network made up of regions that are commonly activated during various types of goal-directed behavior. Regions that are included in the DAN are the inferior parietal cortex, frontal eye fields, supplementary motor area, insula and dorsolateral prefrontal cortices. Some findings suggest that the DMN and the DAN may be anticorrelated,

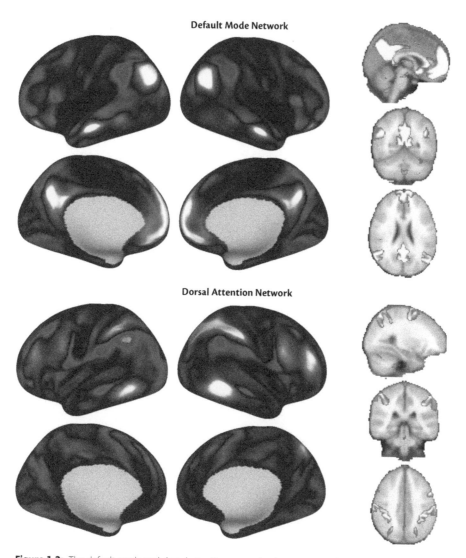

**Figure 1.2:** The default mode and dorsal attention networks shown on a surface view of the brain (left) and on a volumetric view (right). In order to create the surface view, the cortical gray matter ribbon is inflated so that all of the cortical surface (including sulci) can be viewed at once. The top two surface views in each panel show the brain viewed from the left and right side, and the bottom two surface views show a medial view of the brain. For the volumetric images on the right, the most representative sagittal, coronal, and horizontal planes are shown. This figure is showing networks identified using independent component analysis performed on data from the Human Connectome Project (discussed further in Section 1.5).

although these results may, in part, be driven by preprocessing choices. This is discussed in more detail in Chapter 3.

Other commonly described networks include multiple distinguishable visual networks (including dorsal and ventral visual networks), auditory networks, and sensorimotor networks. In addition to the DMN and DAN, additional cognitive networks include salience, executive control, and fronto-parietal networks.

It is important to note that this nomenclature describes a categorization of the brain at a single and somewhat arbitrarily chosen level of granularity. This is to say that these resting state networks form a hierarchy, where networks can be broken down further into yet finer-grained systems (i.e., form "networks within networks"). As such, it is not the case that every area in the brain can be uniquely assigned to one of a set of resting state networks. Indeed, brain regions that are known to have extensive connectivity with many other brain regions, also show functional connectivity with multiple resting state networks.

## 1.3 What can be gained from investigating the resting brain?

There are multiple reasons for choosing to investigate the brain using resting state fMRI. Some of these reasons relate to the types of knowledge that can be gained from studying the brain at rest, whereas others are more pragmatic in nature.

First, resting state fMRI can be used to inform us about the inherent organization and functioning of the brain. Gaining a better understanding of the brain's intrinsic architecture and the level of communication this supports is an important basic neuroscience aim in its own right, and may help us understand how the brain enables complex information processing and rich sets of behaviors, thoughts, and motivations. Likewise, understanding communication in the brain may also help us understand how things go wrong in a variety of different disorders. For example, disorders like attention deficit hyperactivity disorder are thought to be associated with aberrant communication between different regions of the brain.

Additionally, gaining a better understanding of the brain in its basal resting state may be helpful in order to better understand how the brain activates in response to task demands. Currently, task fMRI activation studies commonly rely on the notion that any cognitive process is simply added to anything else that the brain is doing, without affecting any of the other processes (based on the principle of *pure insertion*). This assumption is probably violated in many situations, due to complex interaction between cognitive processes and demands. For example, processes like attention and working memory are involved in even the simplest of tasks. Studying the brain at rest can help to gain a perspective on the variability of spontaneous fluctuations, and how these may be influenced by recent experiences, and by the current cognitive and emotional state of the subject.

In addition to the improved understanding of the basic neuroscience of the brain, resting state fMRI also has great potential to serve as a *biomarker* for mental disorders. A biomarker is something that can be measured accurately and reproducibly, and can therefore serve as an objective indication of the medical state of a person. Biomarkers can be used: (i) as indicators of normal biological processes, (ii) for early detection of for mental disorders, (iii) as markers of disease progression, (iv) as markers of response to treatment, and (v) for creating personalized treatment strategies that are optimized for the patient. No reliable and objective biomarkers are currently available for many mental disorders, but it is hoped that functional connectivity may be used as a biomarker in several of these (such as, for example, depression). Resting state is a particularly promising target for biomarker research because it has many pragmatic benefits (see below), which greatly improve the likelihood of resting state fMRI being used in clinical settings. Additionally, these advantages also mean that it is feasible to obtain enough data to develop normative look-up graphs needed for personalized medicine (similar to the graphs that indicate the distribution of weight for a healthy baby of age 12 months). These advantages are, therefore, very important for what can potentially be gained from studying the resting brain.

The first pragmatic benefit of resting state fMRI is that it does not require a lot of extra equipment beyond the MRI scanner, because there is no need to present the subjects with any information or record any behavioral responses (such as button presses) during the scan. Additionally, the need for expertise of the person acquiring the scan is also reduced, given that no stimulus presentation programming is required and instructions for the participant are minimal. As a result of reduced dependence on equipment and expertise, resting state fMRI is relatively easy to acquire. It also means that resting state fMRI is attractive in the light of data sharing and big data efforts. Additionally, the relative ease of resting state acquisition encourages researchers to replicate their own and other people's findings.

A further pragmatic advantage of investigating the resting brain is the absence of cognitive demands for the subject. Studying subjects at rest is feasible for a large set of subject populations. For example, many clinical populations are unable to perform tasks for a variety of reasons, but may be studied at rest. As a consequence, comparing data across the full lifespan from infancy (or even during prenatal development) to old age is made possible with resting state fMRI. Therefore, the potential of resting state fMRI as a biomarker for early detection and/ or personalized treatment of disorders is vast. Importantly, the relative ease of acquisition and potentially short scan duration means that routine acquisition of resting state fMRI would be feasible in a clinical setting (scan duration is discussed more in Chapter 2). While resting state fMRI is not currently used in clinical practice, this biomarker potential has been a primary driver of the exponential increase of resting state research over the last decade.

While there is much to be gained from studying the resting brain, one common criticism should also be discussed briefly here. Everyone knows intuitively that the brain is not doing "nothing" when we are awake but not engaged in any specific task, and more importantly, we know that the brain can be engaged in a large variety of different processes when "at rest." When the subject is lying in the scanner listening to the scanner sounds during a resting state scan he/she might, for example, be thinking about what to cook for dinner later that night, might be internally rehearsing a skill such as playing the piano, or could be worrying or daydreaming. Studying the brain while it is in this uncontrolled state, that may involve a large variety of processes, is seen as highly problematic by some, because it can be difficult to see how we could learn something about the brain when we are unsure what it is doing in that period. Nevertheless, functional connectivity networks during rest have been shown to be remarkably consistent and can be reliably found across subjects and across studies. These consistent and reliable networks convincingly address one aspect of the criticism outlined above, namely that there appears to be some information represented in the resting brain that can be observed and studied regardless of the subject's cognitive state during rest. However, an important issue that arises from the fact that "rest" is an uncharacterized state (together with inherent limitations of the BOLD signal) is the interpretation of functional connectivity. For example, when we see a change in a resting state network between patients and healthy controls, how can and should we be interpreting this change? Interpretation is a major challenge in resting state fMRI and is discussed in more detail in Chapter 6.

# 1.4  Resting state fMRI signal properties

Functional MRI enables us to record in vivo data from the whole brain at a relatively good spatial and temporal resolution. However, the BOLD signal obtained in fMRI is an indirect, metabolic measure of neural activity mediated by the *hemodynamic response function* (HRF; for an introduction to fMRI please see the primer *Introduction to Neuroimaging Analysis* in this series). As a result, it is necessary to interpret the BOLD signal as a relative, rather than quantitative, measure of activity. Additionally, the BOLD signal is extremely noisy because it is affected by many things other than neural activity, including breathing and cardiac pulsations, and MRI-related artifacts. Therefore, when we show our subject a stimulus, the resulting local increase in neural activity typically only changes the BOLD signal by 1–3% of the baseline BOLD signal. That means that by simply looking at the BOLD images, it is often not possible to "see the activation," that is, it is not possible to distinguish it by eye from the noise.

Many of the challenges faced when analyzing resting state fMRI data result from the large amount of noise and from the indirect nature of the BOLD signal. In resting state fMRI we try to reduce the noise as much as possible with preprocessing, before actually analyzing the data. The reason for this is that functional connectivity methods aim to find similarities in the BOLD signal between two different brain regions, and many types of noise may induce such similarities. Think, for example, about a deep breath or a jolt of movement, these types of artifacts would affect multiple areas of the brain in the same way and could therefore be detected as "functional connectivity." As such, making good preprocessing decisions is extremely important in resting state studies, and many controversies and debates relate to the magnitude and nature of the impact of these preprocessing steps on the results. Commonly adopted preprocessing methods are described and discussed in detail in Chapter 3.

It may be helpful to know that functional connectivity is also commonly described in the literature as correlated *low-frequency fluctuations* (or oscillations) in the BOLD signal. The reason for describing fluctuations as "low frequency" is that the power spectrum of a BOLD timeseries has most power in the low-frequency range (Figure 1.3). Calculating the power spectrum using the *Fourier transform* describes how the variance of the signal is distributed across frequencies; that is, it reflects how much of the changes in signal occur slowly versus more rapidly. The dominance of the low frequencies is not specific to resting state fMRI data; it is an inherent property of the BOLD signal. The reason for this is that the BOLD signal measures blood oxygenation in the active area through the HRF, which takes several seconds to change. Any neural activity is therefore only measured through the veil of the slow HRF, meaning that most of the signal varies relatively slowly over time (which is sometimes referred to by saying that "the HRF acts as a low pass filter").

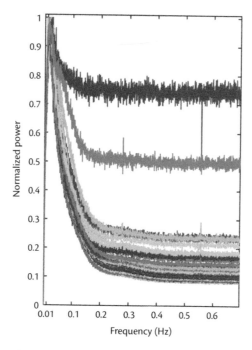

**Figure 1.3:** Fourier transforms can be used to measure the strength of the signal across different frequencies, and the results are visualized as frequency spectra as shown above. The Fourier transforms of 25 resting state networks are shown, and reveal that the resting state BOLD signal is dominated by low-frequency power (i.e., the power is high in the lower frequencies). Two of the networks contain a large amount of noise (red and blue lines), which shows up in the frequency spectrum as relatively high power in higher frequencies (i.e., the spectra have a "raised tail").

Given that much of the power in the BOLD signal occurs at lower frequencies, early functional connectivity studies applied bandpass filtering to resting state data to remove fluctuations over certain frequencies (such as >0.1 Hz) in order to reduce noise (this is discussed in more detail in Chapter 3). However, studies have since shown that information about resting state networks is also present at higher frequencies and, as a result, the term "low-frequency fluctuations" is not seen as often in the recent literature.

Despite the fact that the majority of the power is in the low-frequency range, there is information in the higher frequencies, and it can therefore be beneficial to include the high-frequency data for functional connectivity analyses, instead of throwing it away with bandpass filtering. There is no reason why group differences in functional connectivity (which are most commonly of primary interest in resting state fMRI research) would be limited to the low-frequency range. At a neuronal level, differences between patients and healthy controls may arise from some form of electrophysiological change (for example, ion channels may be altered in patients). To our knowledge, this neuronal change may be reflected in the BOLD signal at any frequency. Therefore, it may be preferable to consider the full range of frequencies when studying resting state fMRI data.

# 1.5 Mapping the human connectome

As described above, a key neuroscientific aim of resting state functional connectivity approaches is to fully understand the intrinsic functional organization of the human brain, and its role in cognition and disease. Therefore, resting state fMRI is an important part of research into human connectomics. The principle goal of *connectomics* is to achieve a comprehensive mapping of brain connectivity across all scales, including neural microscale and systems level macroscale. Given the properties of the BOLD signal, resting state fMRI research is well-suited to study the macroscale connectome, including whole-brain connectivity.

In the age of big data, several large-scale data collection and data sharing efforts have emerged. While it is beyond the scope of this work to cover all of these in detail, several major projects will briefly be mentioned. The *Human Connectome Project* (HCP; http://www.humanconnectome. org) provides MRI data (including resting state and task fMRI, diffusion imaging, and structural scans), as well as extensive behavioral and epidemiological data from 1200 subjects, obtained from family groups. The HCP has resulted in several methodological advances in the fields of both acquisition and analysis of resting state fMRI data, and some of these will be discussed further in later chapters. Another study of note is the UK Biobank Imaging study, which is currently the biggest of all, as it will obtain data on lifestyle, environment, genetics, and multiple multimodal imaging measures, including resting state, from 100,000 subjects. A further project particularly aimed at studying the development of the connectome, is the Developing Human Connectome Project (dHCP), which includes imaging, clinical, behavioral, and genetic data from babies obtained in utero during pregnancy, and in early life (up to 44 weeks post-conception). Another big data sharing effort is fronted by the 1000 functional connectomes project powered by the International NeuroImaging Data-sharing Initiative (INDI), which includes the Autism Brain Imaging Data Exchange (ABIDE). These freely available large collections of data provide an extremely valuable resource for the neuroimaging community and play an important role in advancing our understanding of the human connectome.

## SUMMARY

- The BOLD signal measured in fMRI reflects summation of the synchronized post-synaptic activity (which can be measured as local field potentials).

- Spontaneous BOLD fluctuations measured when participants are resting are correlated across brain regions in a way that reflects the intrinsic functional architecture of the brain.

- Generally speaking, functional connectivity analyses on resting state fMRI aim to examine the relationship between BOLD signals obtained from spatially separate regions of the brain.

- Studying the resting brain can provide information about the intrinsic network structure of the brain, and has the potential to serve as a biomarker for mental disorders.

## FURTHER READING

■ Biswal, B., Yetkin, F.Z., Haughton, V.M., & Hyde, J.S. (1995). Functional connectivity in the motor cortex of resting human brain using echo-planar MRI. *Magnetic Resonance in Medicine, 34*(4), 537–541. Available at: http://www.ncbi.nlm.nih.gov/pubmed/8524021.

    ▨ This is the first paper to show that resting state functional connectivity matches task-based activation patterns.

■ Castellanos, F.X., Di Martino, A., Craddock, R.C., Mehta, A.D., & Milham, M.P. (2013). Clinical applications of the functional connectome. *NeuroImage, 80*, 527–540. Available at: http://doi.org/10.1016/j.neuroimage.2013.04.083.

    ▨ A review of the potential of resting state fMRI as a biomarker, including a discussion of important obstacles.

■ Cole, D.M., Smith, S.M., & Beckmann, C.F. (2010). Advances and pitfalls in the analysis and interpretation of resting-state FMRI data. *Frontiers in Systems Neuroscience, 4*, 8. Available at: https://doi.org/10.3389/fnsys.2010.00008.

    ▨ A useful overview of the field of resting-state fMRI functional connectivity.

■ Jenkinson, M. & Chappell, M. *Introduction to Neuroimaging Analysis.*

    ▨ The introduction primer for this series of neuroimaging primers provides more information about MRI.

■ Smith, S.M., Fox, P.T., Miller, K.L., Glahn, D.C., Fox, P.M., Mackay, C.E., et al. (2009). Correspondence of the brain's functional architecture during activation and rest. *Proceedings of the National Academy of Sciences of the United States of America, 106*(31), 13040–13045. Available at: http://doi.org/10.1073/pnas.0905267106.

    ▨ A relatively early paper summarizing common ICA networks. These networks are available online and are sometimes used as literature masks for functional connectivity analyses (such as dual regression analysis, discussed further in Chapter 4).

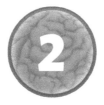

# Data Acquisition

Acquiring resting state fMRI data may sound relatively straightforward, but it nevertheless is useful to be well informed about the options available for acquisition. The amount of structured noise in BOLD data is one of the main challenges in resting state fMRI analysis, and making well-informed decisions when acquiring the data can make a big difference to the results. This chapter covers basic scanning parameters, such as repetition time, as well as different sequence options that are popular in resting state fMRI. Finally, protocol decisions are covered, such as scan duration, and eyes open or closed, as well as how to deal with motion.

Regardless of what sequences and parameters are used for data acquisition (and how often these have been used successfully in the past in your laboratory or department), it is always a good idea to run at least one full pilot subject all the way through to the analysis. This can be useful to highlight any problems in the practicalities of scanning, the quality and coverage of the scan in regions that are of particular interest, and the analysis pipeline. During the acquisition of the full study, it is still advisable to visually check the data of each subject once it has been acquired (i.e., check your data regularly, and do not wait until the end of the study). Data quality could change after the pilot due to hardware replacements, incorrect shimming, subject movement, and many other reasons (for example, a hairclip may get stuck in the bore causing gradient spikes unbeknown to the operators). Some examples of accidental bad data acquisitions are shown in Figure 2.1. Some form of artifact is not uncommon and, therefore, it is very important to visually ensure data quality regularly during your study. If you notice any artifacts in your data, get in touch with the local radiographer, physicist, or analysis expert to get help resolving the problem.

## 2.1 Repetition time, voxel size, and coverage

The most commonly used sequences for acquiring resting state fMRI data are based on echo planar imaging (EPI), and the important scanning parameters that need to be set are

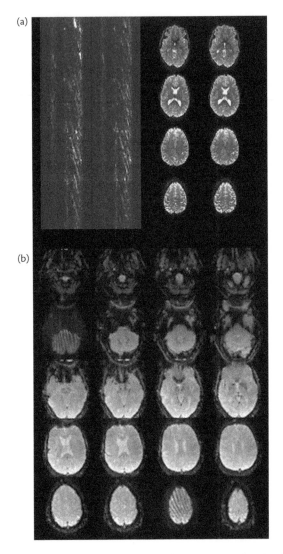

**Figure 2.1:** Examples of data acquisition with artifacts. (a) The shimming failed in this example image on the left; once shimming was corrected the image on the right was acquired. (b) Intermittent gradient spiking problem can be seen in some of the slices; this results from unwanted electrical discharges in the scanner room (potential causes of which include the scanner hardware, metal items, such as a paperclip, lodged in the bore, light bulbs in the scanner room, subject clothing, etc.).

the *repetition time (TR)*, *voxel size*, and *coverage*. A single image of the brain (one volume) is obtained by sequentially acquiring images of all of the slices that cover the brain. For these sequences, the TR is the amount of time it takes to acquire a single whole-brain volume (i.e., the TR controls the temporal resolution). Voxels are three-dimensional pixels, and the size of the voxels therefore determines the spatial resolution of the data. The spatial coverage determines whether data from the whole brain is recorded during the scan or just from a part of the brain. Previous work has shown that resting state networks can be identified robustly across a range of scanning parameters, so the exact choice of these is unlikely to be crucial. Nonetheless, there are some trade-offs and general recommendations that will be briefly mentioned.

First, given that we are typically interested in whole-brain networks in resting state fMRI data, it is often a good idea to make sure the coverage includes the whole brain. Whole-brain coverage is also desirable in light of data-sharing efforts and large multicentre consortium projects. In order to achieve whole-brain coverage in a large proportion of the population without unnecessarily adding extra slices or increasing the voxel size, it is beneficial to orient the scan plane away from the feet (see Figure 2.2), to create an angle of 16 degrees from horizontal (the line between the anterior and posterior commissure; please see Further reading for more information). Nonetheless, some specific research questions may well require reduced coverage that does not include the whole brain, for example, in cases where the brain stem is of particular interest or when an especially low TR is required (<0.5 seconds).

Secondly, it might be tempting to opt for small voxel sizes in order to improve spatial specificity. Given that the cortex is very thin and heavily folded, it is beneficial to have relatively small voxels (less than 3 mm), such that the opposite sides of a sulcal fold (which can contain very different functional regions) are mainly measured in separate voxels instead of being averaged into a single voxel. However, at smaller voxel sizes the amount of signal in each voxel is significantly reduced and the amount of change in the BOLD signal caused by neural activity relative to the overall amount of noise fluctuations in the data is reduced (i.e., lower functional *contrast-to-noise ratio, CNR; and signal-to-noise ratio, SNR*). This relationship between voxel size and SNR is cubic, meaning that an increase in the voxel size from 1 to 2 mm results in an SNR that is eight times better. As a result, voxel sizes that are commonly used in studies performed on a 3-Tesla scanner typically range from 2 to 4 mm. Voxels are three-dimensional objects and can have different sizes for the three different dimensions. It is commonly preferred to opt for *isotropic* voxels for research studies, meaning that voxels are the same size in all three dimensions (cubic). The main reason to have isotropic voxels is to reduce any bias with regard to spatial direction, because non-isotropic voxels would be less sensitive to the heavily-folded structure of the gray matter in certain directions compared with other directions.

Finally, it is useful to be aware that there is a trade-off between temporal and spatial resolution in fMRI. Reducing the slice thickness (one of the dimensions of a voxel) means that more slices are needed to cover the entire brain, and therefore comes at the cost of increasing the TR in order to cover the same area of the brain. This trade-off has been helped by the development of *multiband* accelerated acquisition sequences that have come into regular use since they were adopted in the Human Connectome Project. Multiband acquisitions are discussed in more detail in the next section.

## 2.2 Multiband EPI sequence

In typical echo planar imaging (EPI), data are acquired slice-by-slice, meaning that the data are acquired from one thin slab of the brain, before moving on to the next slab. Modern MRI equipment allows for signals from multiple detector coils to be measured simultaneously. When using a multiband (or simultaneous multislice) accelerated sequence, multiple slices of the brain are acquired at the same time and information from multiple radiofrequency coils is used in order to separate the overlapping images into their separate slices (also called un-aliasing; Figure 2.2). In order to separate signals from different slices, a multi-channel radiofrequency coil, with at least 32 channels, is necessary. The number of slices that are acquired at the same time in a multiband EPI sequence is known as the *multiband factor*, and this factor controls the amount of speed-up that is obtained. While the trade-off between spatial and temporal resolution is still there when using a multiband sequence, it is much less limiting due to the parallel acquisition of multiple slices. For example, it is possible to acquire whole-brain data at 2 mm isotropic spatial resolution with a TR of roughly 1 second when adopting a multiband factor of 6–8 (i.e., acquiring 6 or 8 slices at the same time). In contrast, a typical whole-brain non-multiband EPI acquisition is likely to have 2.5–3.5 mm isotropic voxels and a TR of approximately 3 seconds.

Multiband EPI sequences can be used to reduce the voxel size and/or the TR compared with non-multiband EPI. Researchers typically choose parameters such that the biggest benefit of the multiband acquisition is the reduction in the TR (due to the downsides of extremely small voxel sizes discussed above). There are two main benefits of reducing the TR. The first is that a shorter TR allows sampling of a wider range of frequencies, which improves the sampling of the signal, and can also help with preprocessing, if the TR is fast enough to sample key periodic signals, such as the respiratory cycle. The second advantage of a shorter TR is that increasing the total number of time points in the resting state dataset improves the statistical power in analyses because it increases the *temporal degrees of freedom*, which is discussed further in Chapter 3.

Despite the improvement in spatio-temporal resolution achieved when using a multiband EPI sequence, there are some important differences between regular EPI and multiband EPI

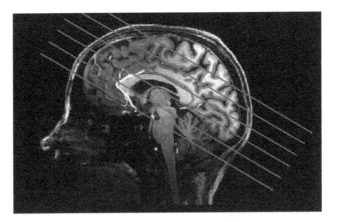

**Figure 2.2:** Using a multiband EPI sequence allows us to push the limits of spatial and temporal resolution. In multiband EPI, data are acquired from multiple slices at once, the multiband factor describes the number of slices acquired at the same time (here the MB factor is six). As described previously, the 16-degree tilt of the field of view helps ensure full brain coverage in a large percentage of the population.

data. First, multiband data can suffer from more artifacts compared with non-multiband EPI. In addition, artifacts that are common to regular and multiband EPI can often look different in multiband EPI due to the multislice acquisition. An example of this is head motion, which can show up as a striped pattern (one line along each simultaneously acquired slice) in multiband EPI, due to the interaction between motion and the slice acquisition pattern. A further effect of multiband EPI acquisition is that the tissue contrast between gray and white matter can be much lower than it is in non-multiband EPI. This reduction in tissue contrast occurs when using short TRs, because the slices are excited in rapid succession, giving tissue less recovery time.

Due to these differences in terms of data acquisition and artifacts, there are some implications for the analysis of multiband data. To address the reduced tissue contrast, it is important to make sure that the sequence also writes out a single-band reference image (a single fMRI volume, often called "SBref"). The purpose of this image is primarily to calibrate the coil profiles to help in the separation of concurrently acquired slices, but this SBref image also has good tissue contrast. The SBref image can subsequently be used for motion correction and for registration to make sure the lack of tissue contrast in the rest of the functional images does not affect these important preprocessing steps. Secondly, due to the sensitivity of multiband EPI to distortions, it is important to apply appropriate shimming during acquisition, and to acquire fieldmaps that can be used later to correct for distortions and aid registration. This is covered in more detail in the section on "Distortion, shimming, and fieldmaps." Finally, head motion can interact with the multi-slice acquisition in multiband data causing striping artifacts, as explained previously. Therefore, it is particularly important to make sure this potential source of noise is dealt with appropriately when preprocessing the data. Chapter 3 will go into preprocessing for resting state fMRI in more detail.

## 2.3  Multi-echo EPI sequence

In a typical EPI sequence a slice in the brain is excited and the signal from this slice is read out after waiting for a certain amount of time (this time gap between excitation and read out is called the *echo time*). The optimal echo time depends on the type of tissue or biological process being examined (as well as the field strength). A common echo time for sensitivity to the BOLD effect in gray matter is 30 ms (at 3 Tesla), and this echo time is typically used for single echo EPI sequences. However, it is possible to add additional signal read outs at shorter echo times without changing the other sequence parameters much, leading to two (or more) images per TR (multi-echo). The data acquired at the shorter echo time will have a considerably lower contribution of BOLD than the read out at the optimal echo time (because there is less BOLD signal to detect when using a shorter echo time), but the noise level remains similar. The advantage of acquiring the second read out at the shorter echo time is that many types of noise found in fMRI are expected to be equally strong regardless of the echo time (i.e., they do not show echo time dependence). This difference in echo time dependence can be used to separate BOLD-like signals from non-BOLD noise and can therefore be useful to "clean up" the data. For this reason, multi-echo sequences are starting to gain popularity in the field of resting state fMRI. Indeed, it is also possible to combine these two acquisition techniques and generate multi-echo multiband data. However, there are still some penalties associated with multi-echo acquisitions, such as an increase in TR compared with multislice acquisitions. Therefore, standard single-echo EPI may well continue to be a better choice overall, as long as artifact removal can be effectively achieved in data preprocessing.

## 2.4 Distortion, shimming, and fieldmaps

When the scanner is empty, the strength of the static magnetic field (often referred to as the $B_0$ field) is relatively homogeneous in the center of the scanner bore, where the head of your subject will be positioned. However, different substances interact with the magnetic field in different ways (particularly brain tissue versus air). Therefore, when your participant lies in the bore of the scanner, the complex structure of different tissues in their head causes inhomogeneities in the magnetic field. These inhomogeneities occur near certain tissue boundaries, for example, near the boundary between the skull and the air sinuses located around the nose. These local changes in the magnetic field strength near tissue boundaries are problematic when acquiring fMRI (EPI) data. The field inhomogeneities interact with the acquisition of the BOLD signal and can therefore lead to signal loss in some areas (*drop out*) or signals ending up in the wrong location (*distortion*); examples of these artifacts are shown in Figure 2.3. These types of imaging artifacts can greatly affect a study and should be thought about carefully during acquisition and analysis.

The MRI scanner is able to optimize the homogeneity of the magnetic field in the bore once the subject is inside. It uses coils inside the bore (called shims) to oppose and ideally cancel out any smooth changes in magnetic field strength induced by various imperfections, including inhomogeneities near the tissue boundaries. These shim coils are essentially little electromagnets that are able to change the magnetic field strength in the bore and, hence, inside the brain. This process of optimizing the magnetic field is called *shimming* and it is important in all MRI acquisitions, and especially for EPI sequences used to acquire BOLD data. Shimming works by measuring the inhomogeneities in the field and then setting the shim coils to approximately counteract these inhomogeneities. Normally, this is done once, although it is possible to shim multiple times (i.e., measuring the field again after changing the field using the coils, to refine the shim). For sequences that are particularly sensitive to magnetic field inhomogeneities, such as multiband EPI, it can be beneficial to shim multiple times.

The aim of shimming is to optimize the homogeneity of the field across the full scan volume of the sequence. However, after shimming there are still artifacts left in problematic areas, such as regions of orbitofrontal cortex, since localized inhomogeneities cannot be canceled by the shimming. Distortions displace some of the data into wrong spatial locations and, therefore, change the shape of the brain. As a result, these distortions are often problematic when trying to register the EPI data to the subject's structural scan. It is therefore advisable to perform distortion correction (which is also called unwarping) as part of the preprocessing pipeline to help achieve the best possible registration (for more information see the primer on *Introduction to Neuroimaging Analysis*). Importantly, distortion correction relies on a fieldmap image that must be obtained during data acquisition. A fieldmap consists of two parts (magnitude and phase image), and essentially contains a map of the remaining magnetic field inhomogeneity after shimming. It only takes about a minute to acquire a fieldmap, and it is important

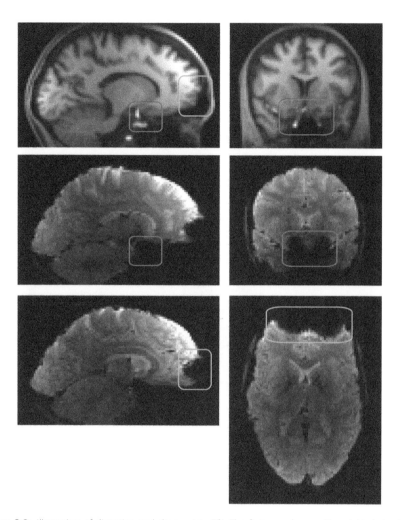

**Figure 2.3:** Illustration of distortion and drop out in EPI. The first row shows a $T_1$-weighted structural image that is resampled and reoriented to match the functional EPI acquisitions shown in the second and third rows, to provide a comparison with the undistorted anatomy. Drop out (signal loss) is prevalent in the inferior frontal lobes, as highlighted by the red boxes (EPI shown in second row, where a large amount of signal is lost within the boxes compared with the $T_1$-weighted structural in the top row). The geometric distortion is highlighted by the blue boxes and is most prominent in the orbitofrontal cortex (it appears as though a bite has been taken out of the frontal cortex in the EPI; third row). Note that the bright parts in the $T_1$-weighted structural image in and near the boxes correspond to blood vessels.

to acquire fieldmaps so that distortion correction can be performed. Note that shimming specifically relates to the location and orientation of the scan volume, and to the position of the subject inside the scanner, so it should be repeated if the subject has moved significantly (for example, came out and went back into the scanner), and also for subsequent sequences with a different size or location of the scan volume. Each time shimming is repeated, new fieldmaps should be acquired because the remaining field inhomogeneities will change after re-shimming.

An alternative to acquiring fieldmaps is to acquire diffusion MRI data in two opposite phase encoding directions (commonly known as "blip-up blip-down"). In the two datasets with reversed phase encoding, the distortions will occur in opposite directions (i.e., areas that are stretched in one phase encode direction become squashed together in the opposite direction). The difference between images acquired in opposite phase encoding directions can be used to estimate a fieldmap directly from the data, avoiding the need for an additional fieldmap acquisition. When adopting a blip-up blip-down acquisitions as an alternative to a fieldmap, it is important to make sure that the scanner does not re-shim in between acquisitions, which can happen automatically (especially when the field of view or the voxel size changes).

## 2.5 Scan duration

How long should a resting state fMRI scan take? This is an important question given that scan time is usually expensive and subject tolerance of lying still in the confined space of a scanner is limited. A highly cited 2010 study by Van Dijk and colleagues showed that 5 minutes of resting state was sufficient to reproducibly identify resting state networks. However, data from the Human Connectome Project has shown that increasing the length of data acquisition (up to 1 hour, 4800 volumes) reduced the noise enough to avoid the need for spatial smoothing of the data, resulting in resting state network maps with improved spatial specificity that map tightly onto the gray matter ribbon. While a 1-hour scan is unlikely to be feasible in many study settings, it may be worth considering increasing the resting state scan time to 10 or 15 minutes to ensure good quality data. The reason for this is that all functional connectivity measures will benefit from the increase in data points, and result in less noisy functional connectivity estimates and better statistics. Specifically, the statistical results obtained from a comparison are related to the square root of the number of time points, so when you decide to acquire double the number of time points, this will improve the statistical result by 41%, assuming that all other aspects influencing the result are kept equal. However, it is important to also consider the perspective of the subject when deciding on the length of scans. For example, if you would like to acquire more than 15 minutes of resting state data, it may be preferable to separate the total scan time into multiple scans of shorter duration to avoid the risk of subjects falling asleep (for example, HCP data is acquired in four scans of 15 minutes).

## 2.6 Eyes open versus eyes closed

Resting state fMRI studies, by definition, usually do not involve many instructions for the participant. Nevertheless, previous work has differentiated between three types of resting state fMRI conditions, namely: (i) eyes closed, (ii) eyes open, and (iii) eyes open with a fixation cross.

There are no large differences between these conditions; that is, very similar networks can be identified regardless of the condition. However, multiple findings have suggested small improvements in reliability of functional connectivity findings when obtained in the condition using eyes open with a fixation cross, compared with the others. It is possible that this improvement in reliability is related to the reduced chance of subjects falling asleep during the scan, when they are instructed to fixate. The effects of sleep and arousal on resting state functional connectivity are discussed more in Chapter 6.

It is worth considering that the cognitive and emotional state of the subject may also influence functional connectivity. Studies have shown that performing a task immediately prior to a resting state scan results in slight changes in certain networks (most notably in networks related to the task). Therefore, resting state fMRI scans are now commonly performed at the start of a scanning session, before any task is performed. Acquiring resting state data first helps with reliability and interpretation of results, and is also beneficial in the light of data sharing. On the other hand, some researchers may be particularly interested in investigating changes in resting state functional connectivity, when subjects are in different emotional or cognitive states, such as to better understand mental disorders like depression and anxiety. For example, it is possible to use a manipulation, such as a stress induction, to study how resting state functional connectivity changes when the same subject is experiencing different levels of state of anxiety. Such state-dependent resting state research is discussed more in Chapter 6.

## 2.7  Motion and physiological confounds

Structured noise in the BOLD data that we acquire is a major obstacle for resting state analysis, and many of the preprocessing steps applied to the data (discussed in detail in the next chapter) are designed to reduce the effects of structured noise. Therefore, it is important to try to minimize noise as much as possible when acquiring the data. For example, padding around the head can be used to reduce motion (while also keeping the subject comfortable). Additionally, for problematic populations such as children or anxious subjects, it may be worthwhile including a training session in a mock-scanner aimed at teaching the subject to reduce head motion prior to acquiring the data. For example, it is possible to set up a mock scanner so that subjects watch a movie that pauses every time their head motion is above a certain threshold. This type of training is a good way to get subjects comfortable with the environment in general, and accustomed to keeping still.

In addition to motion, a further source of structured noise is physiological in nature. The effects of breathing (rate, depth, and volume) and of heart rate include: (i) pulsation in the brain causing local motion, (ii) changes in blood pressure, (iii) changes in blood oxygenation, (iv) changes in arterial carbon dioxide  and (v) changes in vasomotion (i.e., spontaneous changes in the amount of constriction and dilation of blood vessels). Hence, the effects of physiology on resting state BOLD data occur through a variety of complex mechanisms, many of which remain only poorly understood. Some methods that are used to preprocess the data in an attempt to clean up these types of physiological structured noise require the acquisition of physiological data during the scan. For example, the subject's heart rate can be recorded using a pulse oximeter that clips onto a finger, and data on the subject's breathing can be obtained using respiratory bellows (a little belt that goes around the rib cage; also referred to as a pneumatic belt). If your scanner is equipped with a pulse oximeter and bellows, and systems that write out this information for use in preprocessing, it is generally advisable to acquire concurrent physiological data during scanning. These measurements can subsequently be used to help clean up the physiological noise from the data, which is one of the preprocessing options discussed in Chapter 3.

## SUMMARY

- It is useful to be aware of the trade-offs between temporal resolution (TR) and spatial resolution (voxel size + coverage), in order to make informed choices before acquiring data.
- Advanced EPI sequences are available, such as multiband EPI (which acquires multiple slices at the same time to improve spatial and/or temporal resolution), and multi-echo EPI (which acquires multiple images at different echo times to help disambiguate signal from noise).
- Distortions occur near certain tissue boundaries as a result of inhomogeneities in the magnetic field. Shimming is useful to reduce large-scale distortions, but not localized ones. Acquiring fieldmaps is beneficial to be able to apply distortion correction during preprocessing and correct for localized distortions.
- Resting state scans can be short, but longer scans (10 minutes or more) yield better functional connectivity estimates and improved statistics.
- It may be helpful to instruct subjects to keep their eyes open and fixate on a cross shown on the screen to avoid them falling asleep.
- Structured noise resulting from motion, breathing, and heart rate play an important role in resting state fMRI, and should be reduced where possible.

## FURTHER READING

- Huettel, S.A., Song, A.W., and McCarthy, G. (2014). *Functional Magnetic Resonance Imaging* Sinauer Associates Inc., Sunderland, MA.
    - Although quite heavily focused on task fMRI studies, the discussion of physics and acquisition is relevant to resting state fMRI.
- Mennes, M., Jenkinson, M., Valabregue, R., Buitelaar, J.K., Beckmann, C., & Smith, S. (2014). Optimizing full-brain coverage in human brain MRI through population distributions of brain size. *NeuroImage*, *98*, 513–520. Available at: https://doi.org/10.1016/j.neuroimage.2014.04.030.
    - Study suggesting that a 16-degree angle is beneficial for whole brain coverage, as mentioned in Section 2.1.

■ Van Dijk, K.R.A., Hedden, T., Venkataraman, A., Evans, K.C., Lazar, S.W., & Buckner, R.L. (2010). Intrinsic functional connectivity as a tool for human connectomics: theory, properties, and optimization. *Journal of Neurophysiology, 103*(1), 297–321.

  ▫ Study identifying the minimum resting state scan length, as mentioned in Section 2.5. Although it is advisable to consider longer scan times (10–15 minutes) to improve functional connectivity estimates.

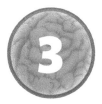

# Data Preprocessing

Once the resting state fMRI data have been acquired and have undergone some form of quality control (such as visually checking the images), the first stage of data analysis is common to all types of resting state studies and involves preprocessing of the data. The main aim of preprocessing is to prepare the resting state data for subsequent functional connectivity analysis by reducing the influence of artifacts and other types of structured noise.

In order to perform functional connectivity analysis, it is extremely important to remove as much structured noise from the data as possible. As discussed in Chapter 1, structured noise can strongly influence any functional connectivity analysis and, if not dealt with appropriately, it is possible for such noise sources to drive your findings. Data preprocessing steps for noise reduction fall into two broad categories. First, there are several noise-reduction steps that are used commonly in any functional MRI research and are not specific to resting state (such as high-pass filtering, spatial smoothing, and motion correction). These steps are covered briefly in Section 3.2 on "Conventional preprocessing steps." Second, additional noise-reduction is essential for any resting state fMRI study due to the risk of structured noise driving the findings. Therefore, the majority of this chapter covers noise-reduction approaches that have been specifically designed to minimize structured noise in resting state functional connectivity studies.

In order to perform a group analysis, it is also important to ensure that we are comparing the same brain regions across subjects. Several preprocessing steps aim to achieve this, including motion correction, registration from functional (echo planar imaging, EPI) to structural ($T_1$) space, registration (or normalization) from structural to standard space, and distortion correction. These preprocessing steps are common to most types of MRI research (including diffusion and task studies), and are therefore only covered briefly in Section 3.2 on "Conventional preprocessing steps."

This chapter starts with a brief introduction to the types of structured noise that affect resting state fMRI, followed by a short discussion of conventional preprocessing steps that are not specific to functional connectivity research. The rest of this chapter will be spent on the explanation of different methods designed specifically to minimize structured noise in resting state fMRI data. For any resting state fMRI study it is essential to include conventional preprocessing steps, and it is also strongly advised to consider using the additional noise-reduction methods covered in this chapter. These additional methods are aimed at addressing the noise-related challenges that are more specific to resting state fMRI. Each of the noise-reduction methods have advantages and disadvantages, which are discussed in each of the sections. Some noise-reduction methods are more common practice, while others were developed and used in early resting state studies, but are infrequently applied in more recent studies, and yet others are somewhat controversial in nature. We should also point out that noise-reduction is an active field that is seeing ongoing research and the development of novel techniques. An overview of steps in a resting state preprocessing pipeline can be found in Figure 3.1, and each of the steps is discussed further in this chapter.

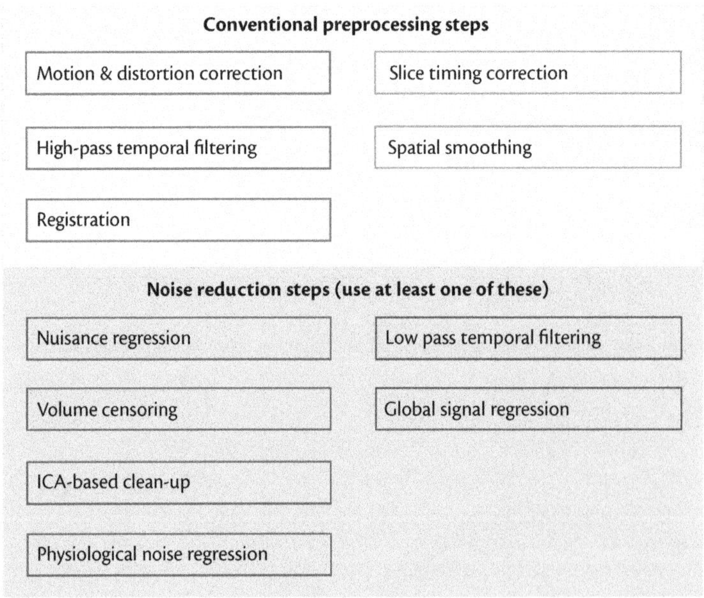

**Conventional preprocessing steps**

| Motion & distortion correction | Slice timing correction |
| High-pass temporal filtering | Spatial smoothing |
| Registration | |

**Noise reduction steps (use at least one of these)**

| Nuisance regression | Low pass temporal filtering |
| Volume censoring | Global signal regression |
| ICA-based clean-up | |
| Physiological noise regression | |

**Figure 3.1:** Overview of preprocessing stages. On the yellow background (top) are conventional preprocessing steps that are common to many types of MRI research including resting state. Of these conventional steps, the ones in the red boxes are always necessary, whereas the ones in the orange boxes are not always required. On the blue background (bottom) are noise-reduction preprocessing steps that have largely been specifically developed for resting state fMRI. The approaches on the left (in bright blue) are more commonly used, whereas the ones on the right (in dark blue) include somewhat dated methods, as well as controversial steps. Each of these preprocessing steps is explained in more detail in this chapter.

# 3.1 Sources of structured noise

There are two primary sources of structured noise in resting state fMRI acquisitions, namely the physiology (i.e., breathing and heartbeat) and movement of the subject while they are in the scanner. Additionally, there may be some artifacts that result from the scanner hardware.

## 3.1.1 Hardware noise

Most types of hardware-induced noise can be substantially reduced or avoided altogether by careful acquisition (including wrap around, radio frequency noise from interfering equipment and ghosting). However, some hardware artifacts are more difficult to avoid and need to be addressed during preprocessing. Examples of the latter are *drift* (which is a very slow change in the baseline BOLD signal over time), distortions, and drop out. Both distortions (seen as warps in the spatial image) and drop out (loss of signal in certain areas, commonly seen in orbitofrontal regions) occur as a result of inhomogeneities in the static magnetic field in the brain, as discussed in Chapter 2. How to address these types of MRI hardware noise is discussed briefly in Section 3.2 on "Conventional preprocessing steps."

## 3.1.2 Head motion

The most problematic cause of structured noise in resting state fMRI data is subject head motion. While head motion can (and should) be reduced by appropriate padding, it is impossible to avoid entirely. Importantly, the amount of head motion often varies across study participants in a way that is related to the research question (e.g., patients often move more than healthy controls) and, therefore, there is a big risk of obtaining resting state fMRI results that are entirely driven by motion. Head motion affects the data in many different ways, which can be largely separated into first- and higher-order motion effects. The first-order effect of motion is simply seen as the spatial misalignment from one volume to the next. It is easy to visualize this first-order effect by watching the raw BOLD data as a movie. In the movie, the image will visibly "dance around" in subjects with more head motion. The first-order effect of motion is corrected using motion correction, which will be discussed briefly in the next section.

Higher-order motion effects, on the other hand, are less intuitive to understand and are much harder to remove from the data. These are effects of head motion that impact subsequent analyses even after the displacements of the individual volumes have been corrected for. Important higher-order motion effects relate to partial volume effects, spin history, and varying field inhomogeneities. *Partial volume* effects result from the fact that voxels at boundaries between tissue types sampled during fMRI are often made up of some combination of gray and white matter, and/or cerebrospinal fluid (CSF), due to the relatively coarse spatial resolution of fMRI. When head motion occurs, the relative contribution of these types of tissue may change because the same voxel is now in a different position in the brain. These partial volume changes can cause secondary changes in the local BOLD signal, which are only approximately corrected by motion correction. In addition, *spin history* effects occur that relate to the fact that the repetition time (TR) in fMRI is too short to allow the magnetic state of the nuclei to completely "forget" about the previous excitation. As long as a region is excited at regular intervals this is not a problem, but when a region moves from one slice to the next due to head motion, the nuclei in that region will be excited slightly earlier or later than expected (i.e., the "history" of the spin excitation differs between nuclei that have not moved between slices and those that have). These spin history effects cause additional changes in the local BOLD signal that cannot be corrected using motion correction. Finally, field inhomogeneities in the static magnetic field occur close to pockets of air, such as around the nasal sinuses, and are corrected for with shimming and fieldmaps (as explained in Chapter 2 and in the next section). When head motion occurs, the field inhomogeneities change, and therefore the shim and fieldmap corrections become suboptimal. As such, complex interactions between motion and drop out can occur, adding localized signal fluctuations. Because movement is such a large contributor to structured noise, and because it is of particular importance if it varies systematically across study participants, many of the preprocessing methods discussed in this chapter aim specifically to reduce the influence of head motion.

### 3.1.3  Physiological noise

In addition to scanner hardware and head motion, a further source of structured noise is physiology, most importantly the cardiac cycle and breathing of the subject. The primary effect of physiological noise on fMRI data is again movement, both in the form of head motion and of pulsatile motion of large arteries, CSF, and surrounding tissue. Taking a breath results in small movements of the chest and abdomen, which often result in a small amount of head motion when the subject is lying down. This is the reason why some degree of head motion is unavoidable when scanning subjects in vivo. Secondly, the changing amount of air in the chest cavity when breathing can change the $B_0$ field and cause bulk susceptibility artifacts.

The cardiac and respiratory cycles are relatively stable (around one heartbeat per second and one breath every 3 seconds), which means that they are easily removable from the data if the sampling frequency is high enough (which is the case, for example, in electroencephalography, EEG). However, the sampling rate (TR) in fMRI is typically too slow to be able to sample these physiological cycles, resulting in aliasing of the signal (i.e., the influence of heartbeat and respiration can end up getting spread out across all frequencies). Hence, in fMRI it is not typically possible to simply filter out the physiological cycles because our sampling is not quick enough. In addition, relative changes in heart rate, and breathing depth and rate also affect things like blood flow, blood oxygenation, blood $CO_2$ levels, and vasodilation. There are some methods that specifically aim to reduce physiological noise, which are covered towards the end of this chapter.

## 3.2  Conventional preprocessing steps

In this section we will briefly explain preprocessing steps that are common to many types of MRI research. More detailed information on these preprocessing steps can be found in the *Introduction to Neuroimaging Analysis* primer in this series.

## 3.2.1  Motion correction

The first preprocessing step that is commonly applied to all fMRI data is motion correction, aimed at correcting the effect of subject head motion in the scanner. This is always necessary because small amounts of head motion are unavoidable. Motion correction works by spatially registering each volume separately to a chosen *reference volume* (i.e., making sure they overlap correctly, thereby removing the gross movement that can be seen in raw BOLD data). The reference volume is usually one of the acquired volumes (either the first or middle volume, depending on the software package that is used). However, sometimes it is better to use an alternative image as the reference; for example, in a multiband sequence the non-saturated image should be used, because it provides better tissue contrast than other volumes (as discussed in Chapter 2). Motion correction applies transformations to each volume such that all resulting volumes are matched up spatially. In addition to aligning the volumes, motion correction also provides outputs of head motion estimates throughout the scan, as a set of *motion parameters*. These motion parameters can be used in later preprocessing stages and are referred to repeatedly in this chapter. There are six motion parameters, three of which describe translations in three directions (left–right, up–down, front–back), and three of which describe rotational movements (pitch, yaw, and roll). Motion correction is essential for all resting state fMRI research, and should always be performed regardless of which additional preprocessing and noise clean-up approaches are used.

## 3.2.2  Slice timing correction

Next, for EPI data, slice timing correction can be applied to resting state fMRI data, but it is not always a requirement. The aim of this step is to correct for the slight difference in the time at which each slice of BOLD data was acquired (i.e., some slices are acquired at the start of the TR, whereas others are acquired later). When the TR of a sequence is, for example, 3 seconds, the difference in slice time acquisition can vary quite a lot and it may be useful to apply slice timing correction. However, with the development of accelerated multiband EPI sequences (Chapter 2), the TR is often closer to 1 second or even less. Given the sluggishness of the hemodynamic response function (Figure 1.1), such small differences in slice time acquisition may have little effect on the analysis. Hence, in studies with fast TRs, it may be beneficial to avoid using slice timing correction because it also has disadvantages, such as the use of interpolation.

Slice timing correction uses *interpolation* in time to slightly shift the BOLD timecourses of voxels in order to account for these small differences in acquisition time. However, interpolation causes a slight temporal smoothing of the data, and therefore results in an unavoidable loss of high-frequency information. Finally, slice timing correction interacts with motion correction and spatial smoothing (discussed in the next section) in ways that are complicated, and typically cannot be corrected fully.

Whether or not to apply slice timing correction should be determined separately for each individual study. This decision should be made based on the TR, and also on the aim of the study and the type of analysis that will be performed after preprocessing (for example, in studies where exact timing is crucial to the hypotheses and methods, slice timing correction may become more important, even for fast TR data).

### 3.2.3 Spatial smoothing

A further step that is commonly applied to various types of (functional-) MRI data in the preprocessing pipeline is to apply some amount of spatial smoothing to the image (also called spatial filtering). Spatial smoothing is achieved by calculating, at each voxel, a weighted average over multiple neighboring voxels and has the effect of blurring the images. The amount of spatial smoothing that is applied is usually defined by the *full-width-half-maximum* (FWHM) of the Gaussian kernel that is used to create the weightings for the averaging (Figure 3.2). The advantage of spatial smoothing is that the averaging helps to reduce the influence of noise. However, the downside of spatial smoothing is that some spatial localization accuracy is lost.

A common rule of thumb is to set the FWHM to 1.5–2 times the size of the voxels in the raw data (i.e., apply spatial smoothing of 4 mm FWHM to data acquired at an isotropic voxel size of 2 mm). However, when deciding on the amount of smoothing to apply to the data, it is also important to consider the size of the regions that you are most interested in. For example,

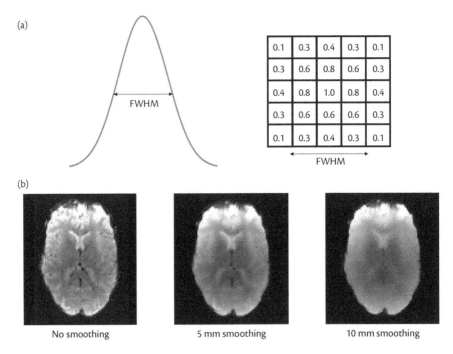

**Figure 3.2:** Spatial smoothing helps with the SNR of the image. (a) The amount of smoothing is based on the smoothing kernel used for the weighted averaging. The properties of the smoothing kernel are defined using the full width half maximum (FWHM); 1D cross section plotted (left) and a 2D cross section shown in the matrix (right), but the kernels used in practice are 3D Gaussians. (b) The effect of spatial smoothing is to blur the image, as shown on these three identical EPI volumes with different amounts of smoothing.

if the aim of a study is to investigate connectivity in the amygdala (a relatively small subcortical structure), then smoothing should be set smaller than the size of the amygdala. In this example, applying too much smoothing would result in blurring the signal too much in the region that is of primary interest for the study.

In EPI datasets with high spatial resolution (i.e., equal to or less than 2.5 mm isotropic voxels) and high temporal resolution (i.e., TR below 1.5 seconds), as well as lengthy timeseries (i.e., at least 10 minutes of acquisition), smoothing is not always necessary. The reason for this is primarily related to the high number of time points available, because more time points leads to a higher number of degrees of freedom (as discussed later in this chapter), which improves the ability to get accurate functional connectivity estimates. However, for lower resolution datasets (in particular, when the number of time points is relatively low), some degree of spatial smoothing may be advantageous.

## 3.2.4 High-pass temporal filtering

The next conventional preprocessing step that is commonly applied to fMRI data is temporal filtering. The aim of temporal filtering is to remove unwanted signal components from the timeseries of each voxel, without removing the signal of interest. Most commonly, fMRI data is high-pass filtered, which means that the very lowest frequencies are removed from the data (when a low cut-off frequency is used this is similar to something that is commonly referred to as "removing the linear trend"; Figure 3.3). The low frequencies that we aim to remove here are

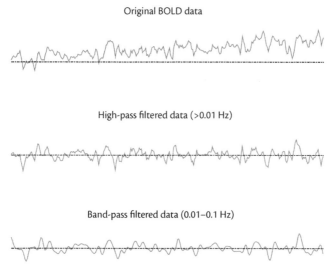

**Figure 3.3:** Effects of temporal filtering. The raw BOLD signal (extracted from the posterior cingulate cortex) shown on the top displays some drift (i.e., the signal amplitude slowly goes up over time). After high-pass filtering this drift has been removed from the data, as shown in the graph in the middle (i.e., the signal at the start of the sequence is no longer lower than the signal at the end of the sequence). On the bottom, the effects of bandpass filtering are shown. Bandpass filtering removes both low and high frequencies from the data, resulting in a smoother timecourse.

ideally lower than the low-frequency fluctuations that dominate the BOLD signal (as described in Chapter 1). The amount of temporal filtering that is applied is typically expressed using a cut-off frequency or a cut-off period. For example, when a high-pass filter with a cut-off of 0.01 Hz (or 100 seconds) is used, this means that any signal fluctuations that vary more slowly than the cut-off will be (entirely or partially) removed (Figure 3.3). Essentially, the aim of high-pass filtering is to remove scanner drift from the data (i.e., changes in the baseline of the BOLD signal that occur slowly over time as a result of the scanner hardware). It is typically advisable to apply high-pass filtering as part of preprocessing. The amount of filtering depends on the data quality; in high quality datasets it is possible to set a higher cut-off period (1000 seconds) in order to remove less and retain more data, whereas lower quality data often use lower cut-off periods (100 seconds) in order to remove more noise. In resting state fMRI, more stringent bandpass temporal filtering is sometimes applied, which is discussed in more detail later in this chapter.

## 3.2.5 Registration

In order to perform group-level analyses (which is usually the aim of any type of fMRI experiment), it is essential to register all subjects to a common "standard" space (as visualized in Figure 3.4). In this section we will briefly discuss the most important aspects of registration. However, registration and the related issues of brain extraction and distortion correction are complex topics, and a more detailed discussion is beyond the scope of this book. Registration, brain extraction, and distortion correction are covered in detail in the introductory primer in this series, *Introduction to Neuroimaging Analysis*.

The *standard space* is a common coordinate system that can be used to describe locations in the brain (common standard spaces that you might have come across are Talairach and Montreal Neurological Institute (MNI) space). Other "spaces" that we often talk about are functional (EPI) and structural ($T_1$) space, which are the native spaces in which the data for each subject are acquired. Importantly, these spaces (functional, structural, and standard) typically have very different image sizes and voxel dimensions, so a voxel in one space will not cover the same region of the brain in the other spaces. The aim of registration is to match up the spatial structure using the images, in order to calculate the transformations between different spaces. These transformations can be used to, for example, place statistical images resulting from a subject-level analysis performed in functional space into standard space to allow group-level comparison. It is also possible to go backwards, for example, in order to transform a region of interest that has been defined in standard space into functional space in order to look at the activation in that region for a specific subject.

Importantly, the brain can be represented in three-dimensional space as it exists in its natural form (also called volumetric space, made up of voxels). However, the gray matter cortex can also be represented on a surface made up of vertices. Registration can be performed in volumetric space or on the cortical surface. Without going into too much detail, the surface representation isolates the ribbon of gray matter that makes up the cortex and either represents this as a flattened sheet, or inflates it until all the gyral folds flatten out, creating an inflated or spherical surface. There is general consensus that registration performed on a surface representation is superior for cortical regions, because in volumetric space two regions that lie on opposite sides of a sulcal fold would be right next to each other (because

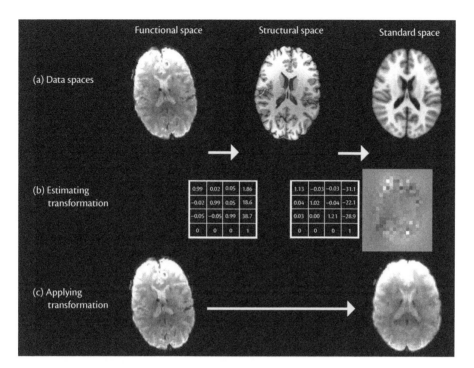

**Figure 3.4:** Registration methods are used to put data from different subjects into the same space so that group comparison can be performed. (a) Different images are acquired in different "spaces." This illustrates a two-stage registration process. (b) The first stage of registration involves estimating the required transformations (which can either be linear matrices, or non-linear warp images). (c) The second step of registration involves applying the transformation in order to resample an image into a different space. The transformations can be combined and applied to resample the EPI functional data into standard space.

of the folding), whereas the surface would accurately reflect the biological distance between the same two regions (because they would separate as a result of flattening or inflation). It has been shown that much better cross-subject alignment of functional areas (and, hence, connectivity) can be achieved through surface-based registration, compared with volumetric registration. Additionally, it is beneficial to perform spatial smoothing on the cortical surface, rather than in volumetric space, to avoid blurring across the sulcal fold. However, surface representations do not capture all the subcortical regions, and these regions are known to play an important role in cognitive and clinical neuroscience. Therefore, it is necessary to work either in volumetric space, or to adopt a hybrid approach that represents the cortex on the surface and subcortical regions as volumes. Such a hybrid approach was developed as part of the Human Connectome Project in the form of a grayordinate system. A *grayordinate* is a gray matter location in the brain that is represented either by a surface vertex for cortical regions or by a volumetric voxel for subcortical regions. We will not discuss surface representations or grayordinates in more detail in this book, but it is important to note that all of the methods described in this book can be applied in either volumetric or surface space (with some adjustments in some cases).

## 3.3 Low-pass temporal filtering

Low-pass filtering is a temporal filtering approach similar to high-pass filtering. However, instead of removing only the lowest frequencies (such as drift), low-pass filtering removes, entirely or partially, the high frequencies above a cut-off frequency (for example, keeping frequencies below 0.1 Hz). Another common term that you might come across is *bandpass filtering*, which is a combination of low- and high-pass filtering (i.e., it keeps the frequencies in between two cut-off frequencies).

Low-pass filtering was common in early resting state functional connectivity analyses, because functional connectivity was considered to be driven by low-frequency oscillations. Therefore, high-frequency BOLD data was thought to only contain noise fluctuations and, as such, it would be preferable to remove frequencies above approximately 0.1 Hz from the data (Figure 3.3). However, it has since been shown that spatial structure, which strongly resembles resting state networks, exists in high-frequency BOLD data, suggesting that the higher frequencies do contain useable signals. Additionally, alternative and more advanced methods for noise-reduction have since been developed, many of which are discussed later. As a result, while it is still an option to use low-pass filtering for noise-reduction purposes, it is no longer seen as an essential step to study resting state fluctuations and is not often used anymore (although as described in Section 3.2, high-pass filtering should be performed to remove drift).

## 3.4 Nuisance regression

A commonly adopted method to reduce the influence of structured noise in resting state fMRI is nuisance regression. In nuisance regression, a set of timecourses are defined that are thought to reflect the variance in the data from different sources of structured noise. These timecourses are called the *nuisance regressors*, and the variances associated with these timecourses are removed from the data using a multiple linear regression (please see the "General Statistics Box: Multiple Linear Regression Analysis (with the GLM)" at the end of this chapter for more details). The signal that remains after the regression (the *residuals*) are then used for further functional connectivity analyses. Timecourses that are included as nuisance regressors often reflect motion, and also BOLD fluctuations from non-gray matter tissues, such as white matter and CSF, as described in more detail later in this chapter.

Many of the subsequent methods discussed in the rest of this chapter are specific versions of nuisance regression, including global signal regression, physiological noise regression, and even some versions of more complex approaches, such as censoring and independent component analysis (ICA). However, in this section we will introduce nuisance regression in the most simple and traditional way. The regression approaches that are explained in this and subsequent sections rely on understanding the multiple linear regression approach (and the concept of residuals), so if you are not familiar with this you may want to take a look at the "General Statistics Box" that can be found at the end of this chapter.

The most commonly used nuisance regressors are the motion parameters (also called realignment parameters), that are estimated during motion correction. There are six motion parameters in total, three for displacement (in the x, y and z directions; also called translations), and three for rotations (pitch, yaw, and roll). Nuisance regression often includes 6, 12, or 24 motion regressors by applying various non-linear transformations to the six parameters that are estimated from the data. For example, a set of 24 motion regressors can include the motion parameters of the current volume, the difference of the motion parameters for the current volume and the volume before it, and the squares of both of these sets of parameters, resulting in a total of 24 nuisance regressors.

In addition to motion parameters, other signals can be derived from the data and used in nuisance regression. For example, one common approach is to extract timeseries representing CSF and white matter (WM). The rationale for including CSF and WM regressors is that fluctuations in these timeseries would not be neuronal in nature (given that it is derived from non-gray matter regions). Instead, it is thought that CSF and WM timeseries are likely to reflect structured noise, such as physiological pulsations (although it is possible that WM timeseries may contain fluctuations from veins that are correlated with neural gray matter BOLD signals). Extracting CSF and WM timeseries can be done by using a segmentation approach in order to obtain a mask of both the CSF and WM, and extracting the mean timeseries from each tissue type by averaging within these masks. Prior to extracting the timeseries, the masks are sometimes eroded (shrunk) to ensure that no boundary voxels are included, because these boundary voxels may contain some gray matter.

The advantages of nuisance regression are that it does not require any additional data acquisition (i.e., the regressors can be estimated using the data), and that it is easy and quick to implement. However, there are two important drawbacks to the nuisance regression approach. Most importantly, because it is based on a linear regression, nuisance regression cannot remove many of the complex secondary effects of motion that were described earlier in this chapter (which are highly complex and non-linear in nature). Secondly, it is important to note that the motion parameters are estimated from the data and are therefore only as good as the accuracy of the algorithm used for motion correction. Due to these drawbacks, the general consensus is that nuisance regression by itself is not sufficient to remove the effect of structured noise prior to functional connectivity analysis. It should therefore only be used in combination with one of the other methods described in this chapter.

## 3.5 Global signal regression

Global signal regression is a specific version of nuisance regression. Obtaining the global signal involves averaging the timeseries across all voxels in the brain, in order to obtain a single average regressor of BOLD fluctuations. This "global" timeseries can then be removed using linear regression (please see the "General Statistics Box" at the end of this chapter for more details). There are two slightly different ways to calculate the "global signal," such that you can either average across all tissue types, including CSF and white matter (which is commonly thought of as the *global signal*), or you can average across the gray matter only (sometimes referred to as the global gray matter signal). In practice, these two averages are typically highly correlated, and the difference between using these two version of the global signal is minimal (especially if nuisance regression of white matter and CSF signals is also adopted).

Importantly, there has been a lot of controversy around global signal regression. Proponents have shown that global signal regression successfully reduces the influence of structured noise on measures of functional connectivity, arguing that it is a straightforward and effective noise-reduction method. However, there are several important negative effects from performing global signal regression. Firstly, because the global signal is calculated using all voxels, it contains a combination of both signal and noise fluctuations. Therefore, global signal regression removes (by definition) some amount of signal from the data. Secondly, removing variability associated with the global signal also changes the connectivity structure across the brain. Specifically, global signal regression introduces a shift in the distribution of functional connectivity values. Importantly, this means that the connectivity between some regions shifts from being zero or positive before global signal regression, to being negative after global signal regression. Hence, global signal regression has been shown to induce negative correlations between brain regions. Given that functional connectivity is the main measure of interest in resting state research, this introduction of negative correlations is an important disadvantage of global signal regression. Due to these unresolved controversies, the use of global signal regression is currently an open debate.

## 3.6  Physiological noise regression

In order to remove physiological noise resulting from cardiac and respiratory fluctuations, it is possible to acquire ongoing physiological measurements while the subject is lying in the scanner. More information about acquiring the physiological data can be found in Chapter 2. These physiological measures can be used during data preprocessing to create regressors that reflect physiological fluctuations. For example, physiological measurements can be used to estimate the phase of both the cardiac and the respiratory cycle, as well as respiration volume and heart rate variability. These regressors (containing one value per acquired volume) can be removed from the data in the same way as nuisance regression (i.e., by taking the residuals from a multiple linear regression). The physiological noise regressors are typically created separately for each slice in order to account for the difference in the timing of each slice that was acquired.

Physiological noise regression is useful for situations when the brain regions that are of primary interest are more likely to be affected by physiological fluctuations as a result of their location in the brain (i.e., inferior regions and those that are close to arteries or veins). Examples of such high-risk brain regions include the brainstem and insula. Additional high-risk brain regions include the anterior cingulate and amygdala, which play a role in psychological processes, such as anxiety, and are therefore strongly associated with physiological responses (to threatening stimuli). Nevertheless, there has been a decline in the use of physiological noise regression over recent years. The most likely reason for this decline is the development of other approaches that perform well and do not require any specific data acquisition (such as independent component analysis, which is discussed in Section 3.8).

# 3.7 Volume censoring

In order to fully remove all primary and secondary effects of motion, one option is to entirely remove the volumes acquired at time points when the subject moved during the scan (Figure 3.5). This approach of removing time points (volumes) from the data entirely is referred to as *volume censoring* (also often called *scrubbing*, *spike removal*, *despiking*, or *spike regression* when the identified volumes are regressed out of the data using a GLM approach, instead of removing the time points altogether). In order to determine movement time points that are to be removed, volume censoring applies a threshold to a measure of movement. *Frame-wise displacement* (FD) is commonly used as the measure of movement, and is calculated by combining the six motion parameters estimated during motion correction into a single measure of displacement (usually by averaging the individual voxel displacements over a brain mask or spherical region of interest (ROI)). There are slight differences in the implementation of FD calculations across platforms; however, all FD measures are strongly correlated so the exact implementation is not important (although the exact values can differ, so it is important to use a threshold value that is related to the specific FD calculation). Volume censoring works by simply removing volumes at time points where the FD was higher than the threshold. Often several volumes just before and just after the peak in FD are also removed to account for effects that might carry over from one TR to the next (such as spin history). Of course, the threshold applied to the frame-wise displacement crucially determines the extent of the clean-up achieved with volume censoring. Thresholds that are commonly used for volume censoring are FD > 0.5 mm (more lenient) or FD > 0.2 mm (more stringent). The relevant implementation of the frame-wise displacement for these suggested thresholds is that by Power and colleagues.

Different measures can also be used to threshold the data and determine which volumes should be removed. A common alternative to frame-wise displacement is known as *DVARS*, which is calculated from the BOLD dataset of a subject (rather than from the motion parameters obtained from the BOLD data). DVARS is an estimate of how much the BOLD signal intensity changes from one time point to the next, averaged across all voxels in the brain. Normally, BOLD data changes relatively smoothly over time due to the hemodynamic response function, so big jumps in the signal are indicative of a noisy volume. DVARS is sensitive to many other types of artifacts in addition to motion.

Volume censoring is effective for removing the effects of motion from resting state fMRI data (including both first-order and higher-order effects) and is a popular noise-reduction approach. However, it is useful to be aware of a few drawbacks of volume censoring. First, the amount of data that is removed in volume censoring is often relatively high (between 20% and 60% of all volumes), meaning that there is a large reduction in the temporal degrees of freedom of the data. The implication of this reduction in degrees of freedom is that the statistical power is reduced (as explained in the "General Statistics Box: Multiple Linear Regression Analysis (with the GLM)" at the end of this chapter). This means that the estimate of functional connectivity becomes more noisy when it is calculated using fewer volumes. Importantly, the number of volumes that are removed varies across subjects as a function of how much the subjects moved. Therefore, the accuracy of the functional connectivity measure estimated within each subject is lower in subjects who moved more, compared with subjects who moved less. When the amount of movement is different between study groups (i.e., between patients and healthy controls) it is possible that this can introduce a

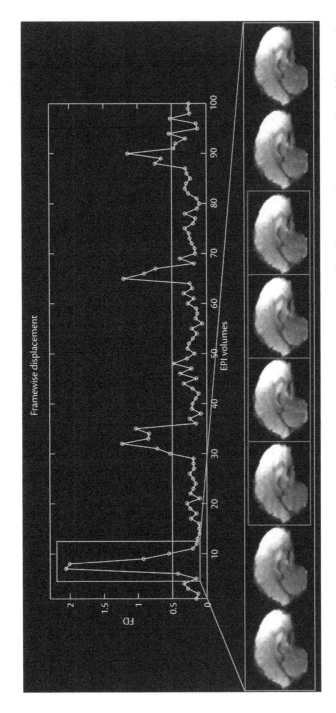

**Figure 3.5:** Volumes with a framewise displacement above a predetermined threshold are removed from the data in volume censoring. Here, eight consecutive EPI volumes (that have undergone conventional preprocessing steps only) are shown reflecting the points in the FD graph highlighted with the green rectangle. The middle four volumes exceed the threshold of 0.5 and are to be removed from the data (indicated by the red boxes).

bias in the group analysis of interest. It is possible to address this issue by making sure that all subjects end up with the same number of volumes (i.e., matching all subjects to the subject with the most volumes removed). However, this may not be the most cost-effective use of scan time, as it would involve removing a large amount of "good" data. Additionally, one would have to think carefully about the pattern used to remove the extra time points that do not exceed the set threshold. Related to the latter comment, a further disadvantage of volume censoring is that the removal of time points disrupts the autocorrelation structure that is present in continuously acquired resting state BOLD data. Disrupting the temporal structure of the data is also problematic in relation to temporal filtering of the data, and may be undesirable when the temporal fluctuations in functional connectivity are of interest to the study (i.e., for dynamic functional connectivity analyses, which are discussed in more detail in Chapter 5). Given that the temporal structure in the data is changed when performing volume censoring, it is also important to consider the order in which different preprocessing steps are performed and how censoring can affect previous stages. For example, temporal filtering should be performed after volume censoring, because the process of removing volumes from the data will change the frequencies present in the data.

To summarize, volume censoring can be an effective method for reducing structured noise from resting state fMRI data, depending on how it is implemented. Therefore, volume censoring is relatively common in resting state fMRI. However, there are other noise reduction methods that may be more flexible, and an example of this is discussed in the next section.

## 3.8  Independent component analysis

Independent component analysis (ICA) is a method that can be used to decompose a whole-brain resting state BOLD dataset into a set of spatially-structured components (Figure 3.6). These components are typically a mixture that contains some components that represent neuronal signal and some components that represent structured noise. Therefore, ICA can be used for clean-up purposes by identifying the noise components and removing these from the data. Note that ICA can also be performed at the group-level to identify large scale resting state networks and group-ICA is covered in Chapter 4, along with a more detailed explanation of how ICA works. The remainder of this section focuses on using single-subject ICA for noise-reduction.

When using ICA for noise-reduction, it should be applied separately to data acquired from each subject (and each run) after conventional preprocessing steps (i.e., motion correction, slice timing correction if used, temporal filtering, and spatial smoothing if used) have been applied. The output from single-subject ICA is a set of components, each of which is described by a spatial map and a timecourse. The number of components that should be extracted can be estimated automatically based on the data, as explained in more detail in Chapter 4. Once ICA has been run to estimate the components, the next step for ICA-based cleanup is to label each of the components as either signal or noise (*classification* of the components). This can be done manually, based on inspecting each of the components, or the labeling can be done using one of the available automated or semi-automated ICA classification methods. Several example signal and noise components are shown in Figure 3.6. The remainder of this chapter

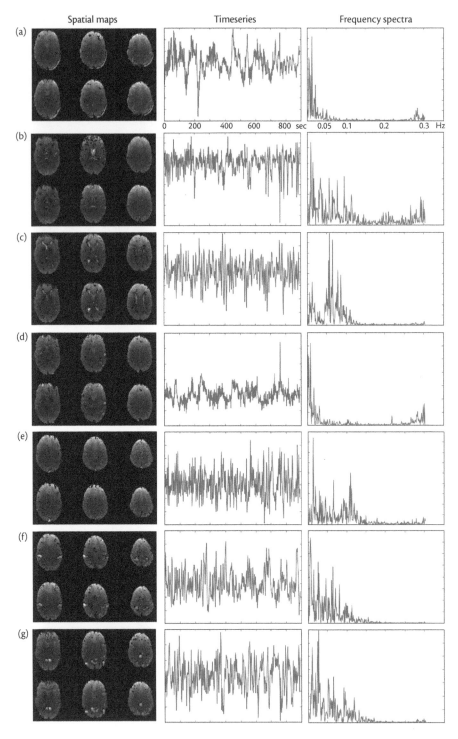

**Figure 3.6:** Examples of noise and signal components from a single-subject ICA: (a) Motion noise component; (b) CSF noise component; (c) white matter noise component; (d) susceptibility motion noise component; (e) sagittal sinus vein noise component; (f) motor signal component; (g) DMN signal component.

provides some guidelines for manual classification, and also introduces a couple of automated classification methods.

Once the components have all been labeled as either signal or noise, the last step is to perform a regression analysis to remove the variance associated with the components labeled as noise from the data. There are two options for removing the noise ICA components from the data, and they are typically known as "aggressive" and "non-aggressive." The aggressive approach is similar to nuisance regression described in Section 3.4, and removes all of the variance explained by the timeseries of the noise components from the data (using multiple linear regression; see "General Statistics Box: Multiple Linear Regression Analysis (with the GLM)" at the end of this chapter). This aggressive approach will lead to the removal of all of the variance that can be explained by the timecourses, even if some of that variance is shared with signal components. The alternative, non-aggressive approach is to only remove the variance that is unique to the noise components and keep in any variance that might be related to signals of interest. That is, it keeps variance that is shared between components labeled as noise relative to components that are not clearly identifiable as being noise, and thus could contain signal. By taking into account the spatial maps and timecourses of the noise components, the regression does not fully remove all variance expressed by the noise timecourse, but only the part of the variance that is not correlated (i.e., shared) with non-noise components. In order to preserve signal as much as possible, the "non-aggressive" approach is typically preferable, because it effectively treats signals as innocent until proven guilty.

## 3.8.1 Guidelines for manually classifying components

Manual inspection and labeling of components is considered the gold standard classification method and is often necessary. For example, some of the semi-automated methods described below require a training set of manually-labeled data, and even when using a fully automated classification approach, it is essential to check the results manually in at least a subset of subjects to ensure accuracy. Additionally, in smaller studies, or when working with difficult populations, it may be preferable to label all data manually. When you visually inspect ICA components for classification, it is important to examine all three pieces of information that are available: the spatial map, the timecourse, and the frequency spectrum of the timecourse, which should all be taken into consideration for every component before coming to a decision.

In terms of the spatial maps, signal components are characterized by a relatively low number of relatively large, contiguous clusters. Additionally, spatial maps should primarily overlap with the gray matter, and peak "activations" should be located within the gray matter. Spatial maps that primarily overlap white matter, CSF, or that show a characteristic ringing around the brain (motion), indicate that the component is noise. In addition to these spatial characteristics, signal components have timeseries that are typically relatively stable with no sudden isolated spikes (such as the spike seen in Figure 3.6d towards the end of the timeseries) and no changes in the oscillation pattern, whereas noise timeseries can often show such spikes or changes over time. Finally, the power spectrum of a signal timeseries should primarily show power in the low-frequency range (below 0.1 Hz), due to the characteristics of the BOLD signal (as discussed in Chapter 1).

While the characteristics described above can be used to identify obvious noise components relatively easily, some noise components appear very similar to signal components in one or two of the three pieces of information. Hence, some components can have signal-like timecourses and/or spectra, yet the spatial map may show that it does not overlap with gray matter (e.g., sagittal sinuses and susceptibility artifacts in regions sensitive to drop out). Additionally, it is possible that a component contains a mixture of signal and noise, which is often reflected in all three pieces of information.

When classifying ICA components for clean-up, it is important to keep in mind that the aim is always to preserve all of the signal present in the dataset. Therefore, carefully consider all three pieces of information in order to pick up clear indications of noise, but when the components may contain a mixture, or when it is not clear whether it is signal or noise take a conservative approach, and do not label these components as noise. Finally, it is useful to note that a large number of the components that are extracted typically consist of noise (70–90% of all extracted components). Additionally, it is common for many of the components ranked first (based on the variance explained) not to contain any signal components.

---

*Example box:* **Single subject ICA**

To get a better feel for the types of noise that exist in a typical dataset, it is useful to have a look at the ICA components that are extracted from a single-subject ICA dataset. On the primer website you will find a set of single subject ICA components. Please use the guidelines described in this chapter to manually classify a set of components into three classes: signal, noise, or unknown (for components that are a mixture or components that are unclear). Once you have labeled the components manually, you will compare your classification to semi-automated labels determined by running the FSL tool called FIX (FMRIB's ICA-based Xnoisefier).

The aim of this example is to get a better feeling for the types of noise present in fMRI data, and to gain some experience with recognizing different ICA signal and noise components.

---

### 3.8.2 Methods for automated component classification

A variety of ICA classification methods that are either fully automated or semi-automated have also been developed. A few specific ones are briefly discussed here, although various other approaches exist. One classification method, called FIX, has gained popularity since its use in the Human Connectome Project. FIX works by extracting a set of 180 features that each represent an aspect of the spatial map, timeseries, or frequency spectrum from the ICA-derived components. These features are used to calculate a score for each component, which reflects how likely it is that the component is signal. A threshold is then applied to these scores to obtain the classification. For example, components with scores lower than 20 may be classified as noise components. The features that FIX uses are similar to the ones suggested above for manually labeling components (such as ringing around the head, high-frequency power, etc.).

Before FIX can be applied, it needs to be trained on data that has been manually classified. This means that you need to feed in the ICA components together with the correct noise or signal labels, so that the FIX algorithm can "learn" how to combine the features into the correct scores. Therefore, at least 10 runs (that represent all the different types of subject groups and runs/conditions that your study may include) should be manually labeled in order to train the FIX algorithm. Importantly, the features used in FIX are sensitive to the acquisition parameters (TR, voxel size, coverage, run length), and to the preprocessing parameters (smoothing, high-pass filtering). Therefore, if FIX has been trained on a dataset in which these parameters are substantially different from a new dataset, it is important to re-train it. While FIX achieves high accuracies for preserving signal and for removing noise from the data, it can be time- consuming to create the manually-labeled training data that is required.

One alternative to FIX that will be briefly discuss here is called ICA-AROMA, which is similar to FIX, because it also uses spatial and temporal features to determine whether an ICA-derived component is signal or noise. However, ICA-AROMA adopts a much simpler approach by using only four features (as opposed to the 180 features used in FIX). As a result, ICA-AROMA does not require any training and can be applied to any dataset without the need to manually label some of the data to train the algorithm. Another advantage of ICA-AROMA, due to the small number of features, is that it only removes components that most people would classify as noise, and can therefore be considered to be a bit more objective compared with FIX. One potential drawback of ICA-AROMA is that it primarily aims to remove components that reflect subject motion from the data. As a result, noise components resulting from non-motion sources are often not labeled as noise and, therefore, not removed from the data. In general, the recommendation is to use FIX when you will be acquiring a lot of data using the same sequence and preprocessing, because in this case it is worthwhile manually labelling some training data, and because it removes both motion and non-motion noise. However, ICA-AROMA may be a preferable approach for smaller-scale studies.

## 3.8.3 Advantages and disadvantages of ICA-based clean-up

The most important advantage of ICA-based clean-up for resting state fMRI is that it is a data-driven method that identifies structure in the BOLD dataset. Therefore, ICA is able to detect noise components from a wide variety of sources, including first- and higher-order motion effects, as well as noise induced by physiology and MRI artifacts. Compared with volume censoring, ICA is able to retain the temporal structure of the data, and generally removes less of the "good" data. ICA-based clean-up has been shown to perform well and is one of the most commonly adopted methods. However, it is useful to be aware of some of the drawbacks of ICA. First, the ability of ICA to successfully separate signal and noise components relies on the temporal (and spatial) resolution of the data. Specifically, components are separated better in datasets that contain more time points. As a result, it can be more challenging to identify pure noise components in relatively low quality data with short acquisitions. Additionally, the ICA clean-up critically depends on the classification of ICA components into signal and noise. There can be some differences in the way different people may label components and also between different automated classification methods (and thresholds). To address these issues it is possible to obtain classifications from multiple raters to assess agreement, and it is certainly advisable to manually verify the classifications obtained from automated methods in at least a subset of subjects, including some subjects with very high and very low motion. In summary, ICA is a popular method that can be used to successfully remove structured noise caused by motion, physiology, and hardware sources from resting state data.

---

*General statistics box:* Multiple linear regression analysis (with the GLM)

This box contains a brief introduction to the concept of a multiple linear regression analysis, because this is the approach that is used to achieve a few key processing steps in this book, namely:

1. During preprocessing, noise clean-up is often achieved using multiple regression (as described earlier in Chapter 3).
2. Dual regression analysis (described in Chapter 4) involves two multiple regression analyses.
3. Cross-subject group-level analysis of functional connectivity data (regardless of the specific method used) typically involves the use of the General Linear Model (which implements a multiple linear regression analysis). The GLM is referred to throughout Chapters 4 and 5 as the main approach to perform cross-subject group-level analyses.

In this box, we will provide a brief introduction to multiple linear regression and the GLM. Given that it is extremely useful to understand multiple regression and the GLM well, we would advise you to read the further information that is available on the primer website: Short Introduction to the General Linear Model for Neuroimaging, especially if you are new to neuroimaging or the GLM.

The general aim of a regression analysis is to create a model that describes some of the signals seen in the data. The model is created by the researcher and is typically made up of several *regressors*, which are the independent variables (also called explanatory variables). These regressors can either describe variance in the data that we are interested in (i.e., the BOLD activation pattern we expect to see in a task fMRI experiment), or it can describe variance in the data that is not interesting and that we would like to remove (such as the nuisance regressors for clean-up of fMRI data described earlier). The dependent variable of a regression analysis is typically either the BOLD resting state data from a single subject or a set of estimated parameter maps across multiple subjects. The latter case will be discussed later in this box, so for now we will assume that the dependent variable for the multiple regression is a preprocessed BOLD dataset from a single subject.

When performing a multiple regression analysis, you are finding the linear combination of the regressors that results in a timeseries that is the "best fit" to the data (i.e., that is most similar and explains as much of the variance in the data as possible). The output of a multiple regression analysis is a *beta* value ($\beta$; also called a parameter estimate or an effect size) for each of the regressors that were included in the model. Each beta value represents how much its associated regressor contributed to the overall linear combination of regressors that was the best fit for the data.

In neuroimaging, the GLM is normally used to analyze whole-brain data, which contains at least tens of thousands of voxels. For each of these voxels, the BOLD signal is measured at every TR, meaning that we have a timeseries of BOLD data at each voxel. When we apply a multiple linear regression analysis (or GLM) to an fMRI dataset, the regression is therefore performed separately for each voxel timeseries, called a voxel-wise analysis (i.e., for each separate analysis the dependent variable is the timeseries from a different voxel). This is also called a *mass univariate analysis*, which simply means that the same analysis is performed many times ("mass"), and is performed separately for every voxel in the brain ("univariate," as opposed to a multivariate analysis, which would take all voxels into account in the same analysis). Therefore, the "best fit" depends on the timeseries of each voxel, and the beta values are different for every voxel. The result of a whole-brain multiple regression analysis is a set of whole brain maps of beta values (one map for each regressor). Each map contains one beta value per voxel, as estimated from the multiple linear regression analysis performed for the BOLD timeseries at that voxel. In Figure 3.7, this would result in two maps, one for $\beta_1$ and one for $\beta_2$.

## Residuals

In addition to estimating the beta values, it is also possible to calculate the *residuals* (also called residual noise or residual errors), which are just the difference between the data and the best fit of the model. The residuals can be calculated by subtracting the sum of each regressor multiplied by its beta value from the data, and the residuals contain the variability that is left over in the data; that is, the variability that could not be explained by any of the regressors entered into the model. Many of the noise reduction approaches discussed in this chapter are descriptions of different methods for creating regressors that explain some of the structured noise seen in fMRI data. Hence, many of the approaches discussed in this chapter work by performing a multiple regression analysis and calculating the residuals. These residuals contain the leftover BOLD data after removing the structured noise, and are therefore the "cleaned up" version of the data that is subsequently used for functional connectivity analysis.

It is also possible to have a model that includes both regressors that are of interest (signal regressors) and nuisance regressors that are aimed at explaining some structure noise variance (noise regressors). This is commonly the case in task fMRI, and can also occur when using the GLM for group-level analyses. In this case, the presence of the noise regressors means that the betas estimated for the signal regressors will be adjusted for variance explained by the noise regressors without the need to calculate the residuals first. This is explained a little bit more in the context of group-level analyses at the end of this box.

## Degrees of freedom

Another aspect of multiple regression is the degrees of freedom. The degrees of freedom is equal to the number of observations (i.e., the number of time points in the BOLD data, or the number of subjects in a group analysis), minus the number of things we would like to

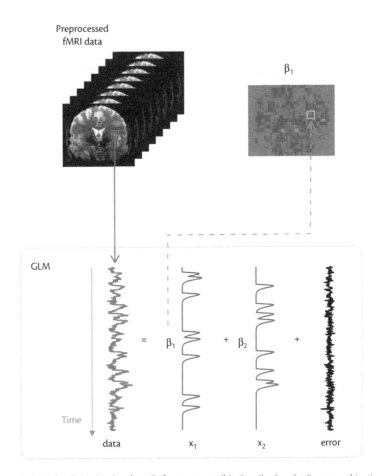

Preprocessed
fMRI data

$\beta_1$

GLM

$=$    $\beta_1$    $+$    $\beta_2$    $+$

Time

data    $x_1$    $x_2$    error

**Figure 3.7:** In the GLM, the data (usually from one voxel) is described as the linear combination of a model (X) containing a set of regressors ($X_1$ and $X_2$). One beta value (representing an amplitude) is calculated for each of the regressors included in the model (i.e., $\hat{\beta}_1$ for $X_1$ and $\hat{\beta}_2$ for $X_2$), and what is left over is the error (i.e., the residuals). This is typically done for all voxels separately, known as a voxelwise analysis, and the results (beta values, or probabilities based on them) are stored, displayed, and possibly analyzed further in the form of voxelwise maps (images, as shown for $\beta_1$ in the top right.).

estimate (i.e., the number of regressors). To get some intuition for what this means imagine that, in order to maintain a healthy weight, you give yourself a lunchtime "constraint": you want to make sure that the average number of calories you consume at lunchtime across any one week (7 days) is 600 Kcal. During the holiday season, you go out for lunch with friends most days and indulge in high calorie options. However, when the last day of the week comes around, you are stuck with a very small plain salad in order to make sure you don't exceed your 600 Kcal average. In this example, you had six degrees of lunch-freedom, because you were free to choose whatever you wanted for 6 of the 7 days. If you had decided that you should average 600 Kcal across the entire month (instead of just across 7 days), then you would have had more degrees of lunch-freedom (i.e., you would have been free to choose whatever you wanted for more days). However, if you put on additional lunch constraints (such as avoiding meat at least 3 days a week), then you would end up reducing your degrees of lunch-freedom further in order to meet the additional constraints. The same happens in a multiple regression analysis; for every parameter that we want to estimate (every constraint we put on our lunch), we lose one degree of freedom.

The number of degrees of freedom is important because it affects the accuracy with which we can estimate the betas for our model. If a multiple regression analysis has a small number of degrees of freedom (i.e., the number of regressors is not much lower than the number of available time points, or than the number of subjects in a group analysis), then the betas cannot be estimated well. When performing a statistical test on the betas, the resulting $p$-value is also related to the degrees of freedom, in a way that reflects this decrease in accuracy. If the degrees of freedom is small, then the effect size needed to pass significance will need to be larger, whereas smaller effect sizes are sufficient to pass significance thresholding if the degrees of freedom are larger. This is the reason why it is often beneficial to increase the scan time or number of subjects in order to increase our degrees of freedom and improve the accuracy of our functional connectivity estimates.

Degrees of freedom are not only relevant for multiple regression analyses; they play a role in any situation where we are estimating one or more value(s) from the data. Therefore, degrees of freedom are relevant to all of the functional connectivity methods discussed in Chapters 4 and 5. Importantly, some functional connectivity methods require more degrees of freedom than others (for example, partial correlation requires more degrees of freedom than full correlation, as discussed in Section 5.4).

## Temporal filtering

When performing a multiple linear regression it is important to ensure that the same temporal filtering that has already been applied to the BOLD data is also applied to the regressors before performing nuisance regression (or any other type of multiple regression). This is an example of the general principle that any operation applied to the data should also be applied to the regressors in order for the model to match (i.e., what you do to one side of the modeling equation—the data—you also need to do to the other side—the regressors). Failing to apply the appropriate filtering to the regressors can actually cause new "noise" to be introduced into the residual data after the regression. This is an easy step to forget and it is often not clearly described in the methods sections of many resting state articles. Nevertheless, it is very important, so remember to make sure that the same frequencies are filtered out of both the data and the regressors prior to running nuisance regression. Note that it is also possible to perform a version of temporal filtering on the BOLD data by including a set of sinusoidal regressors into the GLM model, which is implemented in some software packages (such as Statistical Parametric Mapping (SPM)).

## GLM for group analysis

So far it has been assumed that the dependent variable in the multiple regression is a resting state BOLD dataset from one subject (i.e., this is the data that we are fitting our model to).

However, it is also common that the dependent variable is a set of functional connectivity maps from a group of subjects. Many of the functional connectivity methods discussed in Chapters 4 and 5 result in a functional connectivity map that contains connectivity estimates for each voxel (or for each pair of regions). One (or several) of these functional connectivity maps are typically obtained for each subject, and it is often of interest to perform a group-level analysis to compare these maps across subjects. The most commonly used framework for a group-level analysis is the GLM, which is the same as a multiple linear regression analysis. When using a GLM to perform a group-level analysis, the regressors that make up the model (in a GLM, the set of regressors is also called the "design" or *"design matrix"*—the "X" in Figure 3.7) should each contain one value per subject, and can be used to describe the relationships between subjects. For example, in a patient versus control set-up one of the regressors can contain a value of one for each patient and a value of zero for each control, and a second regressor can contain ones for all controls and zeros for all patients. This GLM can be applied to estimate the means within the patient and control groups, as well as the difference between the two groups, just like an unpaired *t*-test.

Importantly, all of the regressors in a multiple regression analysis are entered into the model at the same time (regardless of whether the analysis is at the group or subject level), and the best fit of each regressor is calculated while taking into account the influence of the other regressors. If there is any *co-linearity* between two of the regressors (i.e., if two regressors are correlated), then this will typically result in a reduction in the beta values calculated from a multiple regression analysis compared with the same analysis, but with one of the co-linear regressors left out. The reason for this is that the variance that is shared between the two regressors (because they are correlated) is split between the two regressors and, hence, the two betas. This type of collinearity is relatively common when performing group-level analyses. For example, if you are interested in comparing the effects of two closely-related aspects of individual differences, such as the self-report questionnaire scores on anxiety and depression scales (which are often highly correlated). Another example is the case in which you may want to control for some uninteresting aspect such as age across subjects, but where age is actually highly correlated with another aspect that you are interested in, such as illness duration or symptom severity. In summary, it is important to carefully consider which regressors to include in your model, and how this might affect the interpretation of the findings.

The GLM is an extremely flexible method for setting up group-level analyses and can be used to perform many types of comparisons, including the sample mean, paired and unpaired *t*-tests, ANOVA, regression against a continuous variable, and many other designs. Due to its versatility, the GLM is adopted for group-level analysis for almost all of the functional connectivity methods described in Chapters 4 and 5. Because of its widespread use in neuroimaging, a comprehensive explanation of the GLM is also available on the primer website (Short Introduction to the General Linear Model for Neuroimaging), and will be covered more extensively in a future primer in the series *Introduction to the General Linear Model*.

## SUMMARY

■ Resting state fMRI data contains a lot of noise resulting from the MRI hardware, subject motion, and subject physiology.

■ The noise is problematic for resting state analyses and needs to be minimized during data preprocessing.

■ Conventional preprocessing steps that are applied to many different types of MRI data include: (i) motion correction, (ii) slice timing correction, (iii) spatial smoothing, (iv) temporal filtering, and (v) registration.

■ For resting state fMRI, additional preprocessing steps are required because functional connectivity analyses look at similarities in the BOLD signal across different brain regions and this is more sensitive to structured noise than other imaging analysis methods.

■ Commonly used additional preprocessing steps include:
   ▪ *Nuisance regression*: variance that can be explained by a set of regressors, including motion parameters, and timeseries extracted from CSF and white matter regions, is removed from the data.
   ▪ *Physiological noise regression*: regressors that explain signals arising from the cardiac and respiratory cycle, and well as heart and breathing rates are calculated using acquired physiological data, and variance that can be explained by these physiological regressors is removed from the data.
   ▪ *Volume censoring*: high motion time points (i.e., when motion is above a predetermined threshold) are entirely removed from the data.
   ▪ *Single subject ICA*: the data are decomposed into components and noise components are identified: variance associated with the noise components is removed from the data.

■ At least one of these additional preprocessing steps should always be used in any resting state fMRI study (in addition to conventional preprocessing steps).

## FURTHER READING

■ Birn, R. M. (2012). The role of physiological noise in resting-state functional connectivity. *NeuroImage*, 62(2), 864–870. Available at: http://doi.org/10.1016/j.neuroimage.2012.01.016.
   ▪ A review paper of physiological noise influences and removal from resting state fMRI data.

■ Bulte, D., & Wartolowska, K. (2016). Monitoring Cardiac and Respiratory Physiology During FMRI. *NeuroImage*. Available at: https://doi.org/10.1016/j.neuroimage.2016.12.001.
   ▪ A paper discussing the impact of physiology on both fMRI and arterial spin labeling datasets.

■ Griffanti, L., Douaud, G., Bijsterbosch, J., Evangelisti, S., Alfaro-Almagro, F., Glasser, M. F., et al. (2016). Hand classification of fMRI ICA noise components. *NeuroImage*. Available at: https://doi.org/10.1016/j.neuroimage.2016.12.036.
  ▪ A paper providing detailed guidelines on how to classify single-subject ICA components into signal and noise for the purpose of data clean-up.
■ Jenkinson, M. & Chappell, M. *Introduction to Neuroimaging Analysis* (the first primer in this series).
  ▪ This volume of the same Primers in Neuroimaging series contains more information about the conventional preprocessing steps that were only briefly covered here.
■ Murphy, K. & Fox, M.D. (2016). Towards a Consensus Regarding Global Signal Regression for Resting State Functional Connectivity MRI. *NeuroImage*. Available at: https://doi.org/10.1016/j.neuroimage.2016.11.052.
  ▪ Review paper with a useful discussion on the benefits and disadvantages of global signal regression.
■ Power, J.D., Schlaggar, B.L., & Petersen, S.E. (2015). Recent progress and outstanding issues in motion correction in resting state fMRI. *NeuroImage*, 105(0), 536–551. Available at: http://doi.org/10.1016/j.neuroimage.2014.10.044.
  ▪ A paper that discusses the problem of subject motion and a large variety of preprocessing methods that aim at reducing motion.

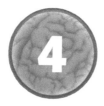

# Voxel-based Connectivity Analyses

After preprocessing, the fMRI resting state data are ready for functional connectivity analysis. As described in chapter 1, the vast majority of methods used to study resting state functional connectivity aim at detecting similarities among distinct regions of the brain, in line with the definition of functional connectivity. There are a wide variety of different connectivity analyses, and new approaches are still being developed. These functional connectivity methods can be broadly divided into voxel-based and node-based methods. The key aspect that voxel-based methods have in common is that they all estimate a functional connectivity value for each voxel in the brain (i.e., they describe functional connectivity in terms of spatially distributed effects). Therefore, regardless of differences in how individual voxel-based methods estimate functional connectivity, all of these methods result in a map (or multiple maps) of the brain containing values for all voxels. This map-based output is the main difference between voxel-based and node-based methods. Commonly used node-based methods will be introduced in detail in chapter 5, while this chapter will describe multiple voxel-based methods that are widely used.

Several commonly adopted voxel-based functional connectivity analyses will be described, including seed-based correlation analysis (SCA), independent component analysis (ICA), fractional amplitude of low-frequency fluctuations (fALFF), and regional homogeneity (ReHo). We will discuss how to calculate each measure at the single subject level, how to perform a group-level analysis to compare the maps across subjects, as well as advantages and disadvantages of each method.

It is helpful to realize that there are no totally "right" or "wrong" functional connectivity approaches. All of the methods discussed in this chapter and in the next chapter are commonly used and play a role in the growing fields of resting state fMRI and connectomics. However, there are more appropriate and less appropriate functional connectivity methods depending on your dataset and your research question. Therefore, the aim of these chapters is to provide a comprehensive overview of the most commonly used approaches, so that you are able to make an informed decision about the most appropriate analysis choice for your research.

While we are aiming to cover a wide range of common methods in these two chapters, there are other methods available and there are novel methods being proposed all the time.

The definition of functional connectivity in chapter 1, together with the discussion of common methods in these two chapters, should provide a good preparation, even if you end up using one of the less common approaches not directly discussed here.

# 4.1  Seed-based correlation analysis

In a seed-based correlation analysis (SCA), one region of interest is chosen that will drive the resulting functional connectivity map. This *region of interest (ROI; also called the seed region)* can be a single voxel, or more commonly a functional region made up of a group of voxels. The aim of a seed-based analysis is to obtain a whole brain map that describes the strength of functional connectivity of each voxel in the brain with the region of interest. Therefore, the resulting map describes the whole brain functional connectivity pattern of the seed region of interest.

Several of the steps that are involved when performing a seed-based analysis are also important steps of node-based analyses, which are discussed more in the next chapter. The reason for this is that node-based methods aim to estimate connectivity between a set of brain regions. The difference between SCA and node-based methods is that SCA defines a single ROI or seed region and looks at functional connectivity of the whole brain with this region, whereas node-based methods define a set of regions in the brain and look at connections between these regions (i.e., node-based methods do not estimate a map of connectivity). Due to the overlap, the discussion of the first two steps of SCA below is relatively short, and refers to sections in the next chapter (there is no need to skip to the next chapter to read these sections at this point, just go through the material in order).

The first step in SCA is to spatially define the seed ROI (which is similar to a "node" in node-based methods). Typically, the seed is a functional region that includes multiple voxels, and defining the region involves determining where the boundaries of the seed region are (i.e., which voxels are included and not included). There are several approaches to ROI definition, including the use of available atlases and data-driven approaches. More detail on different approaches for defining an ROI can be found in chapter 5 (Section 5.2). In general, using a data-driven approach to localize the region and define the boundaries can provide a more accurate estimate of the true functional boundaries in the data compared with atlas-based approaches, and is, therefore, a preferred option.

Once the seed ROI has been defined, the second step in SCA is to extract the BOLD timeseries from the ROI in each subject (Figure 4.1). If the ROI is larger than a single voxel, the BOLD timeseries of the seed region can, for example, be calculated as the mean across voxels for each time point. Timecourse extraction is discussed in more detail in Section 5.3.

Once the ROI timeseries has been extracted, the next step is to calculate the seed-based connectivity map for each subject. To achieve this, the correlation coefficient between the timeseries of voxel A and the timeseries of the seed ROI is calculated, and the resulting correlation is entered into the connectivity map at the location of voxel A. This is repeated for all of the voxels in the brain, resulting in a whole brain connectivity map (Figure 4.1). The resulting

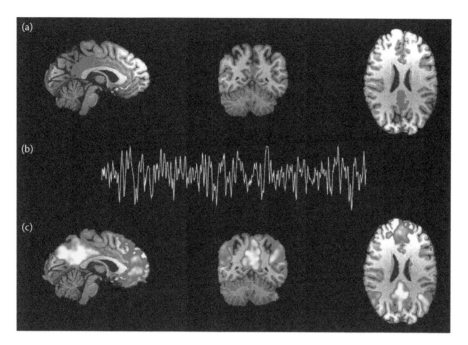

**Figure 4.1:** Results from a seed-based correlation analysis on a single subject. (a) The seed region of interest in the posterior cingulate cortex is shown in blue. (b) The average BOLD timeseries extracted from this region. (c) A thresholded correlation map of all other voxels with this seed timeseries is shown. SCA can be used to find resting state networks such as the DMN, as shown here, depending on the location of the seed.

seed-based connectivity map is obtained for each subject, and these subject maps can be used in subsequent group-level analyses.

Before performing a group-level analysis, the subject-wise correlation maps are often transformed to Z-scores using *Fisher's r-to-Z transformation*. Z-transforming the voxel-wise correlation values changes the range of the numbers, because correlation values range from -1 to +1, whereas Z-values are not bounded by upper or lower limits. Z-transforming the values is often useful for subsequent statistical group comparisons.

The seed-based functional connectivity maps (correlation $r$-values or Z-statistics) that are estimated for each individual subject can subsequently be entered into a group-level analysis. Common group-level questions may be: (i) which brain regions have, on average, the strongest functional connectivity with the seed ROI across all subjects, (ii) in which brain regions does functional connectivity with the seed region differ between two groups, for example, between patients and healthy controls, or iii) in which brain regions does seed-based connectivity vary across subjects in a way that is related to other cross-subject measures such as intelligence or anxiety? Group-level analyses for voxel-based methods are explained at the end of this chapter (Section 4.6).

---

**Example box: Seed-based correlation analysis**

There are multiple steps involved in running a seed-based correlation analysis on a single subject, including:

1. Defining the seed region (using anatomical or functional information).
2. Transforming the seed region into functional space, because it is quite common for the seed to be created in a different space (such as standard space).
3. Extracting the ROI timeseries.
4. Performing the voxel-wise correlation at every voxel relative to the seed timeseries to create the SCA map.
5. Fisher's r-to-Z transformation.

This exercise will take you through some of these steps. The aim of this exercise is to become familiar with some of the practicalities involved in a single subject SCA.

---

### 4.1.1 Advantages and disadvantages of SCA

The main advantage of adopting a seed-based correlation analysis approach is that it addresses a relatively specific question, namely the whole brain connectivity pattern of a chosen region, and how this connectivity pattern might change across subjects. As a result, it is a relatively hypothesis-driven approach compared with other, more data-driven methods discussed later in this chapter (most notably Independent Component Analysis; ICA). Therefore, if your study specifically aims to investigate changes in, for example, amygdala connectivity between patients with an anxiety disorder and healthy controls, then SCA is a good method to consider. Another, more pragmatic advantage of SCA is that it is relatively easy (and fast) to calculate.

An important disadvantage of SCA is that it is limited to the chosen seed, and to the spatial definition of the seed. Hence, you will only be able to study changes in amygdala connectivity if this is your chosen seed region, even though changes in connectivity between two other regions may also occur. More generally, the results of a seed-based correlation analysis only consider one system (i.e., one temporal signal) at a time, even though it is expected that the brain is most likely made up of multiple networks acting simultaneously and potentially with significant spatial overlap with each other. While the interpretation of SCA results is superficially relatively straightforward, the fact that a potentially large set of secondary signals occurring at the same time are being ignored means that SCA findings are likely to represent an oversimplification of the true network dynamics, complicating the interpretation. Additionally, the results of a seed-based analysis are sensitive to the spatial localization of the seed ROI. It has been shown that very different findings can sometimes be obtained when shifting the ROI spatially by only a small amount. This is an important consideration and implies that extreme care should be taken when defining the seed ROI, and also when interpreting the results and comparing different seed-based studies that may investigate the same region, but that use slightly different spatial ROIs.

## 4.2 Independent component analysis

Compared with the relatively hypothesis-driven approach of SCA, independent component analysis (ICA) is at the other end of the spectrum, being a fully data-driven (or "model free"), exploratory data analysis method. ICA is a data-driven, exploratory method that is adopted in a wide variety of fields and applications. The aim of ICA is to decompose a multivariate signal into a set of features that represent some structure that is present in the data (called *components*; see Figure 3.6). Hence, ICA assumes that the observed data is a mixture of multiple underlying components that cannot be directly observed, but that can be separated. An example to understand the concept is being in a room listening to a lecture; you can hear the lecturer's voice, but you might also hear birds singing outside, repetitive banging from the construction noises at the building next door, and perhaps even acquisition noises coming from the MRI scanner in the room below. Therefore, the signal that your ears pick up is a mixture of all these sources, but your brain is able to separate them and pay attention to the lecturer's voice. ICA takes the same approach to resting state fMRI data (although it requires many more data points than just the input from your two ears), and aims to separate the BOLD signal (which is the mixture observed here) into separate underlying components that were combined to create the mixture. Therefore, ICA is by definition a multivariate approach, because it considers all of the data from all voxels at once to find the components, instead of separately analyzing each voxel independently of the others.

When applying ICA, each resulting component is described as a spatial map (which reflects where in the brain a certain signal portion is being detected), and a timeseries (describing how the signal evolved over time). ICA is a linear model, which means that the original dataset can be recreated simply by summing all of the components together (Box 4.1). ICA can be used to extract a set of resting state networks from a dataset, including the default mode network and dorsal attentional network introduced in Chapter 1, as well as many other cognitive, motor and sensory networks. It has been shown that these resting state networks can be found very reliably when using ICA across a wide range of resting state fMRI data acquisition protocols.

---

### Box 4.1:  The ICA model

For those of you who are comfortable with maths, this box provides a slightly more technical introduction to ICA. However, the rest of this chapter does not require that you understand the contents of this box.

Figure 4.2 shows a matrix representation of ICA. The fMRI data on the left hand side contains the BOLD data such that each row represents data from a 3D volume at one time point and each column represents data from all time points at one voxel. The voxels are all reordered and lined up next to each other to create one long row, per time point, that represents the entire three-dimensional brain. After running ICA, this data is unmixed into a set of components that are each described by their own timecourse (that contains the same number of time points as the input data) and a spatial map. One timecourse is extracted for each component (i.e., the number of columns represents the *dimensionality* or *model order*).

For each of the timecourses there is a spatial map, and these are represented in the same way as the input data such that all voxels are lined up in one long row (consisting of the same number of columns, i.e., the same number of voxels, as the input data). The number of rows in the spatial map matrix is the same as the number of columns in the timecourses matrix, and represents the ICA dimensionality (i.e., the number of components).

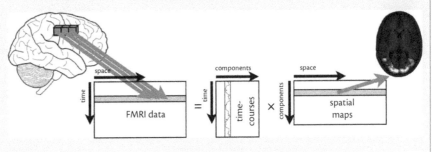

**Figure 4.2:** Matrix algebra description of ICA.

How does ICA identify the components in the dataset? Remember that within the ICA framework we assume that the data we observe was generated by mixing together underlying components (with associated spatial and temporal features), which are not directly observable. In order to identify these components from the data, it is necessary to perform the *unmixing* of the observed BOLD signal (a technical term for this is that we need to *factorize* the data matrix). There are various different ways of unmixing the data, which all use different types of assumptions. ICA looks specifically for components that are maximally independent from one another. *Statistical independence* essentially means that there is no statistical relationship between two derived components (i.e., they are not correlated and they do not have any higher order relationships). When two signals are statistically independent, there is no way to predict signal two based on knowledge about signal one. Take the example of throwing two dice: knowing about the result on one of them does not help you to predict what the value of the second dice might be. In ICA statistical independence is used to "unmix" resting state data into its underlying independent components.

The constraint of independence has to be applied to one of the dimensions of the data, so in the case of resting state fMRI analysis it is possible to choose to either look for signals that are temporally independent (temporal ICA), or to look for signals that are spatially independent (spatial ICA). While both spatial and temporal ICA have been applied to resting state fMRI data to study functional connectivity, by far the most commonly adopted approach is spatial ICA. The reason for this is partly because we usually have many more voxels (up to 100,000 for typical data) than time points (commonly hundreds or in best cases a few thousand per subject), and partly because the underlying signals are much more non-Gaussian in space than in time (see Box 4.2 on How does the ICA "unmixing" work?). When all other things are equal, spatial ICA, therefore, performs better than temporal ICA.

## Box 4.2: How does the ICA "unmixing" work?

In order to estimate the set of independent spatial maps and associated timecourses, it is necessary to use a *cost function* that measures statistical independence. A cost function is a mathematical function that can be optimized in order to find an optimal solution to a problem; in this case, a good set of independent components. One common cost function adopted in the estimation of ICA components is based on the principle of non-Gaussianity. The reason for being interested in non-Gaussianity is because it is known that when signals are combined together to form a mixture, the averaging that is happening to create the mixture causes the distribution of this mixture to be more Gaussian than the distribution of the original signals that went into the mixture (Figure 4.3). This is, in fact, what is predicted by the central limit theorem of statistics, which states that a mixture of distributions tends to be more Gaussian than the underlying parts. We can measure the degree of non-Gaussianity in various ways, and one particularly efficient way is to use *negative entropy*, which measures the non-Gaussianity in a signal by assessing how different the distribution of the signal is from a Gaussian distribution. In summary, by finding the set of components that are maximally non-Gaussian (as measured by negative entropy) it is possible to identify the set of timecourses and independent spatial maps that explain the data.

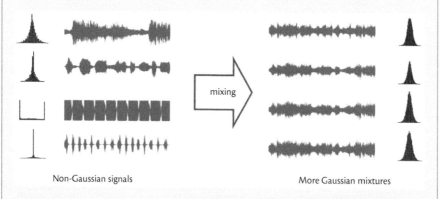

Non-Gaussian signals · mixing · More Gaussian mixtures

**Figure 4.3:** This figure demonstrates how combining signals together results in mixtures that are more Gaussian. In this example, four different sounds (left) are mixed together to create mixtures (right). The distributions of the signals after mixing are much more Gaussian (as seen on the extreme right) than the distributions of the original source signals (extreme left). The principle is the same for ICA applied to resting state data, although we typically optimize non-Gaussianity across space, rather than across time (i.e., the distributions in spatial ICA are the histograms of values over space).

## 4.2.1 Probabilistic ICA and dimensionality

One common problem for data-driven methods such as ICA is the risk of overfitting the data. Ideally, the number of components that are extracted should explain all the "interesting" structure in the data (regardless of whether it is neuronal or artifactual structure). Overfitting occurs when too many components are used to describe very noisy parts of the data, and is, therefore, a common problem in noisy datasets like BOLD fMRI. To avoid overfitting, a probabilistic ICA model can be used, which assumes that the data can be summarized as the component spatial maps and timecourses plus some additional noise.

However, even using a probabilistic ICA model, it is still challenging to determine how many components should be extracted from the data (also called the *model order selection* or the *dimensionality*). It is possible to use the data itself in order to get an estimate of the number of components, by using principal component analysis (PCA). PCA is a *decomposition method* that is similar to ICA, but instead of independence, PCA looks for components that are orthogonal to each other (uncorrelated) and that explain the maximum amount of variance in the data. In practice, PCA is always performed as part of any ICA decomposition in order to reduce the dimensionality of the data. We can use the PCA data reduction step in order to estimate the total number of components that explain the data well. There is a known function that describes how much variance is explained by each subsequent PCA component when the data are purely made up of unstructured white noise, and this function can be used for model order selection. Specifically, we can run PCA on our data and continue to extract components until the next component explains only as much variance as would be expected if the remaining data were made up of unstructured white noise. At that point we can stop and ignore the remaining set of noisy PCA components. ICA is subsequently performed on the dataset that is left over after removing the PCA components associated with the unstructured noise (though structured noise, such as artifacts, will still be left). The number of independent components that will then be extracted is the same as the number of PCA components that were estimated.

In practice, automatic model order estimation is useful to get an idea of the dimensionality of the data. However, as explained below, it is sometimes useful (particularly with multiple-subject group-ICA) to manually set the number of components to a lower number in order to obtain familiar resting state networks that are more consistent with other studies in the literature. When the dimensionality increases, networks like the DMN can start to be split up into several different components. Such split components, although they may well be biologically driven, can make it difficult to reconcile the results with the existing resting state literature, which is why a lower dimensionality is sometimes desirable (particularly for a group-ICA decomposition).

It is worth noting that the order of components extracted using ICA is relatively arbitrary. Therefore, when the same analysis is performed twice on the same dataset, the order of the extracted components can differ. In practice, it is common to apply some post-hoc ordering to the set of extracted components, for example, by ordering these in terms of the amount of uniquely explained variance. However, note that the aim of ICA is to decompose the data into components that are present in the data, therefore, the order of the components is not particularly important.

## 4.2.2  Group-ICA decomposition

ICA can be applied to data from a single subject (or run), as explained in chapter 3, in order to identify and remove noise components. However, ICA can also be used at the group level in order to identify large-scale resting state networks (such as the default mode network), using resting state from a group of subjects. When performing a group-ICA, the inputs are the preprocessed and cleaned resting state BOLD data from all subjects (i.e., the

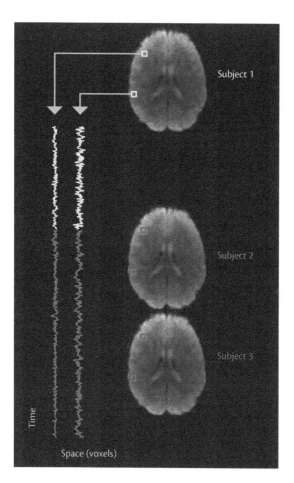

**Figure 4.4:** Group-ICA is performed by combining all the data from the subjects after they have been registered to a standard space. For resting state analysis, the data should be temporally concatenated across subjects for the group-ICA. This means that the data from subject 2 is pasted after the data from subject 1 (and so forth) in order to create one very long dataset. Spatially, each of the voxels are placed next to one another in a long row, in order to end up with a two-dimensional matrix where the columns contain the long, concatenated timeseries and the rows contain information from all voxels in the brain.

components extracted in the single-subject ICA decomposition are not needed for the group-ICA). In order to extract group-level components, it is necessary to combine the data from all subjects. Combining resting state fMRI data for a group-level ICA decomposition is typically done by spatially registering all subjects to a standard space and then *temporally concatenating* the registered datasets from all subjects together. This means that the dataset from subject 2 is pasted after the last time point of the dataset from subject 1 and so on, effectively creating one really long dataset (Figure 4.4). The concatenated dataset from all subjects is then fed into ICA, and components are extracted using data from all subjects. The output from a concatenated group-ICA still contains a set of spatial maps (one per component, representing the group map), and a set of timeseries (a very long timeseries for each component, containing subject 1 first and then subject 2, etc., in order of the concatenation). Another method for running group-ICA is the tensor ICA approach, which combines all subjects in a separate subject-dimension. This approach is preferable if all subjects are expected to have similar timecourses (such as when they are all performing the same task). However, for resting state group-ICA, the temporal concatenation approach should be used.

The result of a group-ICA decomposition is a single group-level spatial map for each component. However, it is often of interest to run statistical analyses to compare components between groups of subjects, for example, in order to ask questions like: are there any changes in the default mode network between patients suffering from depression and healthy control subjects? To address this type of question a further analysis is required in order to calculate subject-specific maps that can be compared, and a commonly used approach for this is a dual regression analysis, which is discussed in the next section.

---

*Example box:* **Group-ICA networks from different datasets**

The results of a group-ICA decomposition can look different depending on the acquisition parameters (such as voxel size and TR), preprocessing steps (for example, whether the data were smoothed or not), and the group size (number of subjects). The same holds true for many other types of functional connectivity analyses. Additionally, the dimensionality of the group-ICA decomposition can typically split up networks in different ways, as described previously. Therefore, it is useful to become familiar with looking at resting state networks obtained from different datasets, different dimensionalities, and also in a variety of different views (e.g., surface versus volumetric visualizations). On the primer website you will find examples of group-ICA networks from different datasets and with different dimensionalities.

The aim of this short example is to show you a set of resting state networks to help you get familiar with recognizing these common networks across a variety of datasets of visualizations.

## 4.2.3  Advantages and disadvantages of ICA

The networks identified in ICA represent regions that show similarity in their timecourses across the period of the scan, which is much like what is done by SCA. Hence, often one of the networks derived from ICA will be similar to the result of a seed-based correlation map found with SCA (Figure 4.1). A major advantage of ICA over SCA is that it is a fully multivariate data-driven approach, which means that ICA estimates the full spatial structure of all of the networks that make up the resting state signal. By decomposing the full dataset into structured components, ICA is able to better differentiate between components that reflect structured noise, and components that reflect networks of interest, and is also better able to distinguish between different networks of interest. In addition, the data-driven nature of ICA also means that it is not sensitive to differences in the definition of the seed ROI, and that ICA is able to describe multiple different resting state networks, rather than only being sensitive to the functional connectivity pattern of the seed region.

When performing an ICA decomposition, there are several important things to take into consideration. Firstly, the dimensionality of the ICA decomposition (i.e., how many networks are extracted) is a factor that plays an important role in the resulting network structure. As explained above, the dimensionality can be estimated from the data, or can be controlled manually. It is important to appreciate that there can be no single "best" dimensionality for the underlying neurophysiology of multiple distributed systems. The reason for this is that it is likely that the hierarchical structure of the brain can be explained at multiple levels of complexity. The dimensionality interacts with interpretation, because networks extracted with ICA can sometimes be split or combined in a way that can make identification of networks in relation to existing literature challenging. Determining an appropriate dimensionality for your study depends on the analysis methods used (higher dimensional ICA decomposition can be used for node-based analyses discussed in the next chapter, whereas lower dimensionality ICA are more common for dual regression analyses), and should also be informed by the literature (it is easier to compare findings if the network structure in different studies is comparable).

A second consideration is that the order of extracted components potentially varies if you run the same analysis again on the same dataset (and even the components themselves may change slightly). The reason for this is that the ICA decomposition involves optimization of a set of parameters, and the result can vary (due to the method used for optimization). This variability is often minor, but it is useful to be aware that the decomposition will not be identical if you run the same analysis again.

Limited spatial overlap between ICA components, resulting from the fact that components are required to be spatially independent, is sometimes considered a disadvantage of ICA. However, some overlap is possible, as a result of the amount of noise in the data. Specifically, if there was very little noise, two partially overlapping components would be spatially correlated and would, therefore, not be allowed as two independent components. However, in the presence of noise, the correlation between two components with a small amount of spatial overlap can go down to zero, and ICA can recover the overlap after thresholding. Nevertheless, the components that are extracted using spatial ICA are still largely non-overlapping. While we do not currently have a complete understanding of the "true" network structure of the resting brain, it is likely that some regions might be part of multiple networks.

# 4.3 Obtaining subject-wise ICA estimates with dual regression

In order to statistically compare ICA components and detect differences in the resting state networks between subjects or groups of subjects, it is necessary to obtain subject-wise component maps. Hence, for each component, you want to obtain one map per subject that describes the component specifically for that subject (Figure 4.5). Perhaps the most obvious option for getting subject maps of ICA components is to perform single-subject ICA on each subject and then match the components to each other post-hoc. However, in practice it is often the case that a network will be described by a single component in one subject, but split into two (or even three) separate components in another subject (i.e., there is a *correspondence problem*). Therefore, there is a big risk that you end up comparing components that are not well-matched, and it would be hard to interpret whether any resulting group differences are truly neuronal in nature, or are driven by some arbitrary difference in the decomposition across subjects. Therefore, a more practical solution is to run a group analysis in order to ensure that the components are the same across all subjects, and then map these group components back to individual subjects. A couple of different approaches are available for obtaining subject maps based on group-ICA components, which are described below.

One approach that has been suggested and applied in order to obtain individual subject maps is called *back-projection*. In this approach, the PCA data reduction step is applied separately to the data from each subject, and the resulting subject-level PCA components are then "projected" onto the group-level ICA unmixing matrix. A projection is simply a way

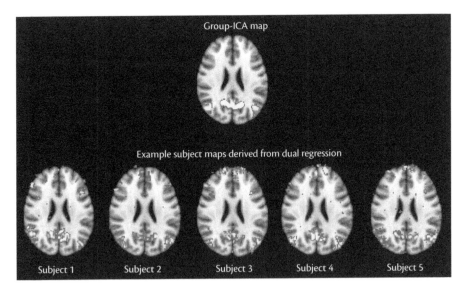

**Figure 4.5:** Dual regression can be used to extract subject-specific maps based on a group-ICA component. The subject maps can then be statistically compared at the group level to detect significant differences.

of remixing the data in terms of the ICA components instead of the PCA components, so it is like asking "how much of each of the PCAs do I need to construct each one of the ICA components?" While this method aims to achieve better correspondence between group and subject maps, it does suffer from some problems resulting from the fact that the PCA dimensionality reduction is performed independently for each subject, which has several implications for the resulting subject maps. Firstly, the subject maps that are obtained may not fully represent all of the differences between subjects, meaning that some of differences between groups (which may be of key interest for the study) can be lost. Secondly, there is no guarantee that the same, consistent information across subjects is retained after the PCA data reduction step. Thirdly, there may be different amounts of subject-specific structured noise for different subjects, which can introduce differences in the PCA dimensionality reduction across subjects, potentially affecting the statistical results (for example, if important between-subject differences are lost in the dimensionality reduction for some subjects, the statistical results may be over optimistic).

An alternative method, *dual regression*, is a common approach to obtaining and comparing subject maps, and this will be explained in more detail below. The dual regression technique uses the group-ICA maps and applies two subsequent regression analyses using the original preprocessed dataset from each subject in order to derive subject-specific maps. As the name suggests, dual regression involves two stages, both of which are multiple regression analyses (general linear models, see the "General Statistics Box: Multiple Linear Regression Analysis (with the GLM)" in chapter 3). The idea behind dual regression is to use the group-ICA maps as a template model of the overall network structure within each subject, and to find the subject-maps that best fit this model.

The two stages of a dual regression analysis are essentially the same as steps two and three of an SCA (i.e., extracting the timeseries, and correlating each voxel against the extracted timeseries). In fact, if you enter a single seed-based ROI map (instead of multiple group-ICA maps) into a dual regression analysis, the results will be identical to performing an SCA. The key difference is that we typically use a set of group-ICA maps as the input for the dual regression analysis. This means that instead of a simple correlation, we are performing multiple regression for both stage 1 and stage 2 of dual regression (this is discussed in more detail below). Another important difference is that the group-ICA maps contain weights for all voxels, whereas a seed region in SCA is typically a binary mask (containing ones within the seed region and zeros in all other areas of the brain).

As explained in Figure 4.6, the first stage of a dual regression analysis is to perform a multiple regression analysis where the group-ICA maps are the spatial regressors (independent variables), and the subject's preprocessed BOLD dataset is the input data (dependent variable). The result of this first stage of dual regression is a set of timecourses (one for each group map) that describe the temporal structure of each component for that subject (similar to the timecourse extraction stage in SCA). Essentially the timecourses contain information on how much each of the components contributed to the overall BOLD signal. These timecourses derived from stage 1 of the dual regression now become the model input for the second regression. Stage 2 involves the second multiple regression analysis, where the temporal regressors obtained from stage 1 (independent variables) are regressed against the same subject's preprocessed BOLD data (dependent variable). The output of stage 2 of dual regression is a set of maps (one for each original group-level ICA component) that describe the network structure based on the data from that subject alone. Together, the outputs from stage 1 and 2 give us subject maps

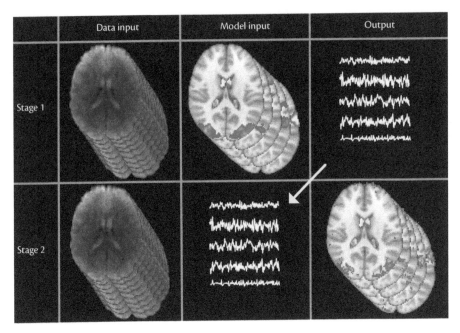

|  | Data input | Model input | Output |
| --- | --- | --- | --- |
| Stage 1 |  |  |  |
| Stage 2 |  |  |  |

**Figure 4.6:** Dual regression is a two-stage process aimed at obtaining component spatial maps for every subject. The data input to the multiple regression analysis is the same in both stages (i.e., the preprocessed BOLD data from one subject). The model input for stage 1 contains the set of ICA components from the group-ICA. The outputs of stage 1 are the subject-specific component timeseries for each group component of interest, and these are used as the model input for stage 2 of the dual regression analysis. The spatial maps that are obtained from stage 2 can be used in a group analysis.

that best fit the group-ICA maps that are used as a starting point. The subject maps can contain either parameter estimates (beta values) or Z-statistics (which have been normalized by the within-subject noise) at every voxel. While either of these types of maps can be used for further group-level analysis, it is the beta maps that are most commonly used.

The outputs from stage 2 of the dual regression (i.e., the subject maps) are subsequently used for between-subject analyses. Specifically, the subject-specific maps can be used for group-level comparisons to study differences in network structure between subjects (which is sometimes called stage 3 of dual regression). For example, you can ask in what regions a certain network might differ in shape or strength between a group of patients and a group of healthy control subjects. Or you can look at individual difference analyses, for example, in what regions of the brain the shape or size of a network varies across subjects in a way that is linked to a cross-subject measure such as disease severity, or mathematical ability. Group-level analysis for voxel-based methods is discussed in more detail in Section 4.6.

It is important for the dual regression approach that each stage involves a *multiple* regression analysis. This means that regressors corresponding to all the components are entered into the model together and the best fit of each regressor is calculated while taking into account the influence of the other regressors (see "General Statistics Box" in chapter 3). Remember that in our case the regressors for stage 1 of the dual regression represent the group-ICA maps. The set of components obtained from a group-ICA fully represent the group data (at least, the part of the group data that was kept after the PCA data reduction step). Group-ICA decomposition commonly results in multiple structured noise components even after performing careful clean-up of the subject data, because some structured noise is only detected by ICA when data from all subjects are analyzed at the same time. Therefore, the timecourses that are the output from the multiple spatial regression (stage 1 of the dual regression) represent the unique signal associated with each component, while the noise components capture confounding, unwanted noise timecourses as long as they are entered into the same multiple regression analysis. For this reason, it often is useful to include all of the components extracted from the group-ICA in the dual regression analysis, even if you are only interested in looking at a few of them in subsequent analyses. This essentially provides another useful way to denoise the single-subject estimates, by using noise components that exist on average at the group level. Further, within the dual regression procedure we go back to the full original timeseries data at both stages of the analysis. This is important to avoid the PCA-bias of back projection methods discussed earlier, and to achieve accurate statistics in any down-stream comparison.

## 4.3.1 Stage 1 timeseries normalization

The timecourse output from stage 1 of the dual regression is often rescaled before using it as the model for stage 2. This normalization involves dividing the timecourse of each component by its standard deviation, which means that the variances of all of the timeseries are the same (set to 1) after rescaling. The advantage of applying this type of normalization is that the subject maps obtained at the end of stage 2 of the dual regression represent both between-subject differences in the shape of the networks, and also in the strength of the networks. For example, if the DMN is twice as strong in subject A than in subject B (in terms of the regression values being twice as large), the dual regression maps will show this difference in "network strength" if this normalization was applied to the timeseries before entering them into the stage 2 regression. If such a normalization has not been applied, the estimated "network strength" (stage 2 output) of the dual regression maps for both subjects would be the same. Without normalization, the timeseries output of stage 1 of the dual regression will reflect this difference in "strength" (i.e., the amplitude of the timeseries will be bigger in subject A than in subject B). When these unnormalized timeseries are used as the regressors in stage 2 of the dual regression, and fit to the datasets of the subjects, the difference in strength is already represented by the regressors and, therefore, the betas in the subject map (stage 2 outputs) will not reflect the difference in strength. However, if rescaling is performed on the timeseries extracted by stage 1, then these timeseries will no longer reflect the difference in strength (i.e., the standard deviation of the timeseries in both subjects A and B will be set to one). When these normalized timeseries are used in stage 2 as regressors and fit to the data of the subjects, the betas in the subject map will now reflect the scaling that is needed so that the normalized timeseries match the subject's data well. Therefore, the betas in the subject map will end up being bigger in subject A compared with subject B, and as a result the maps will reflect the difference in network strength.

In summary, any magnitude differences either end up in the stage 1 outputs (i.e., in the timeseries, if no rescaling is done), or in the stage 2 outputs (i.e., in the spatial maps, if timeseries rescaling is done). Therefore, if you are interested in differences in either shape or amplitude of the networks (which is commonly the case), you should apply stage 1 timeseries normalization.

---

*Example box:* **Visualizing dual regression group analysis results**

The output of a group-level statistical analysis of dual regression maps is a set of whole-brain maps; one for each of the group-level ICA components that were entered into the dual regression analysis and selected for statistical comparison. Each of these result maps should be viewed and interpreted in relation to the relevant group-level ICA component that was entered into the dual regression analysis. It is also possible to perform a number of different statistical tests (e.g., a group difference, or investigating the relationship with a covariate of interest), in which case the outputs include one map for each group-level ICA component and for each separate statistical test in the analysis. On the primer website you will find an example dual regression results folder, as well as instructions to help you navigate through the outputs, and visualize and interpret a set of results. The aim of this example is to help improve your understanding of dual regression and to get experience looking at some results.

---

## 4.3.2 Which group maps to enter into a dual regression analysis?

So far it has been assumed that we are using group-level ICA maps (that were estimated using the data from all of the subjects) as the input to the dual regression. However, the dual regression procedure itself is very generic, and it is possible to enter any set of maps. The three most common inputs to a dual regression analysis are:

1. Group-ICA maps based on subjects from the same dataset (as described above).
2. Template maps that were obtained from past studies (some sets of maps can be freely downloaded).
3. Maps that were obtained from a group-ICA decomposition performed on a set of independent subjects (none of whom are included in the subsequent dual regression and group-level analyses).

All of the steps in the dual regression analysis and group-level comparison of the subject maps are exactly the same regardless of the maps that are fed into stage 1 of the dual regression. There are advantages and disadvantages for each of the three possible inputs described above, and these are discussed in more detail below. Which of these three is preferable for your study critically depends on your research question and study design (especially whether you have an equal number of subjects in all experimental groups).

The advantage of the first option (i.e., group-ICA maps based on all subjects) is that these maps provide the best representation of the structured components that are present in your dataset (including structured noise components). Therefore, this approach is likely to be the most sensitive to detecting any results, partly because the components represent the network structure well, and partly because it is able to model any remaining noise that is identified with group-ICA. One potential downside of this approach is that the group-ICA decomposition may split networks up in a way that is different to the networks described in the literature, which can make comparisons with previous work more challenging. Another potential disadvantage of this approach is that the group-ICA will give a hybrid map that is somewhere between the two (or more) experimental groups included in your study (i.e., for components in which there is a difference between the groups, the group-ICA map does not represent the network in either of the groups very well), which can make interpretation of group difference results challenging. For example, a single region may be part of a network in healthy controls, and may be completely absent from the network in the patient group. The group-ICA map will show that this region is, on average across the two groups, weakly part of the network (because it is an average between the two groups), and the dual regression results will show that there is a significant difference between the two groups in this region. However, coming to the correct interpretation, that the region is there in one group and not in the other group, is difficult based on this information.

A further complication occurs when groups are not equal in size. For example, consider a study that aims to look at the difference between Parkinson's patients and healthy controls, and the dataset includes 20 controls and 80 Parkinson's patients. In this scenario, there are two options for obtaining group-ICA maps. The first is to include all 100 subjects into the group-ICA, and the second option is to include an equal number of subjects from both groups into the group-ICA (i.e., all 20 controls and a subset of 20 Parkinson's patients). For both of these options, the advantages are the same as those described above (i.e., both approaches are able to represent the structure present in the data, including group-level noise). An advantage of the first approach (i.e., including all subjects) is that there is more data available to define the group-ICA maps. However, the resulting group map is more heavily influenced by the larger group, which might result in lower sensitivity to regions that are different in the smaller group. An advantage of the second option (using equal numbers of subjects in both groups) is that the group map might be a more balanced representation across the two groups (especially if the original groups are very unequal in size). However, there may be a statistical bias in this scenario, because the group-ICA maps do not represent all subjects (i.e., those not included in the group-ICA are likely to differ more from the group-ICA components). To circumvent these complications, it is generally preferable to avoid having unequal group sizes to start with. Regardless of whether you have equal or unequal group sizes, the problems with literature compatibility and interpretation described in the previous paragraph still exist.

The second option for inputs to a dual regression analysis is to use *template maps* available in the literature. The advantage of this approach is that it ensures that networks are split in a way that is consistent with the literature and, therefore, allows easy comparison between studies. Furthermore, in the case of uneven group numbers, the use of templates can help to avoid the issues of biases and complexities in interpreting findings that are described above. However, template maps do not represent the structure that is present in the specific dataset as well as a group-ICA performed on the same data (for example, the structure of components may differ as a result of study sample demographics, fMRI acquisition parameters, etc.). In addition, any noise components present at the group level (which are study-specific) are not represented by template maps. Furthermore, some group differences might only be detectable using maps that better represent the structure in the specific dataset, and may, therefore, be missed when using template maps.

The third option is to use group-ICA maps that are obtained from a group of subjects that are independent from the subjects used for subsequent dual regression and group comparison analyses. For example, you may have access to an earlier study performed by your lab and from these subjects it is possible to obtain group-ICA maps that can be used in your more recent Parkinson's study. This approach is similar to using template maps, but can benefit from the fact that there may be a better match between the data driving the group-ICA and the data used for subsequent dual regression analysis. For example, the demographics, acquisition parameters, and preprocessing are likely to be more similar between two studies performed in the same lab. However, maps obtained from a different group of subjects still do not fully represent the structure present in the subjects of interest, and the maps may be relatively noisy if the number of subjects used to drive the group-ICA is small. For this option, it is very important to make sure that none of the subjects included in the group-ICA are also part of subsequent group comparisons. For example, you should not run a group-ICA on subjects from just one of the experimental groups (i.e., just the healthy controls), which are then included in subsequent group comparisons, as this approach introduces a statistical bias and should always be avoided. This bias does not occur when using an independent group of subjects or when using a template map (option two).

In summary, the dual regression approach is flexible and there are a number of different ways to obtain group maps that can be fed into a dual regression analysis. Deciding which of the options described above is best for your study depends on your research question and experimental groups.

## 4.4 Amplitude of low-frequency fluctuations

While most measures of resting state functional connectivity focus on detecting similarities in fluctuations of the BOLD signal between two regions, it is also possible to determine potentially interesting measures within an individual region. For example, it is possible to measure the amplitude of the low-frequency fluctuations (ALFF) for each voxel of the brain. As discussed in chapter 1, the BOLD signal is dominated by low-frequency fluctuations (because of the slow timescale of the hemodynamic response function). Therefore, it is possible to attempt to estimate the neuronal component of the measured BOLD signal in any region by determining how much of the power is in the low-frequency range. It has been shown that this low-frequency amplitude is higher in gray matter than in white matter, and is highest in regions involved in the DMN, such as the posterior cingulate and medial prefrontal cortex. Therefore, ALFF may provide a marker that can be used to highlight brain regions with altered low-frequency amplitudes in groups of patients (for example, in ADHD children) compared with healthy controls.

ALFF is defined as the total power within the frequency range between 0.01 and 0.1 Hz, and is calculated separately for each voxel. In order to calculate ALFF, the Fourier transform of the voxel timeseries is calculated. As explained in chapter 1, the Fourier transform is used to calculate the power spectrum of a timeseries, reflecting how the signal is composed of separate frequencies (i.e., the power at a certain frequency relates to the size of the fluctuations in the timeseries at that frequency). Based on the Fourier transform, ALFF can be calculated by taking the average square root power within the low-frequency range (0.01–0.1 Hz). This measure of ALFF is commonly standardized by dividing it by the global mean ALFF (i.e., the mean calculated across all voxels). Repeating this calculation at each voxel results in a whole brain map of ALFF values for each subject. These subject maps can be entered into a group-level analysis using the GLM framework in the same way as for SCA and dual regression subject maps (Section 4.6).

A normalized version of ALFF was developed when it became apparent that ALFF is sensitive to some types of noise fluctuations, particularly near major arteries and veins as well as near the ventricles and cisterns. The fractional amplitude of low-frequency fluctuations (fALFF) is considered to be more specifically sensitive to low-frequency fluctuations that are neuronal in origin. Fractional ALFF is defined as the total power in the low-frequency range (0.01–0.1 Hz) divided by the total power across the entire (detectable) frequency range for the same voxel. It is calculated by dividing the average square root power in the low-frequency range by the average square root power across all estimated frequencies. Note that bandpass filtering should not be applied prior to fALFF calculation, because the full frequency power spectrum is needed. Group-level analysis using fALFF maps again uses the general linear model to ask questions about, for example, differences between subject groups (see Section 4.6).

### 4.4.1 Advantages and disadvantages of ALFF and fALFF

Both ALFF and fALFF are relatively easy and fast to calculate and result in a summary map of low-frequency power for each subject. However, it is important to note that this method does not measure functional connectivity directly, because it does not look at similarities between separate brain regions (i.e., there is no guarantee that (f)ALFF results are related to functional connectivity). Instead, results from ALFF and fALFF analyses summarize the frequency characteristics of the local BOLD data. As a result, (f)ALFF measures are potentially also more sensitive to non-neuronal confounds from scanner artifacts or physiology compared with other methods discussed in this chapter.

## 4.5 Regional homogeneity

Most resting state fMRI methods investigate functional connectivity across the entire brain and are, therefore, primarily sensitive to long-distance connections (as is the case for SCA and ICA described earlier in this chapter). The next method, however, particularly aims to describe functional connectivity at a local level between neighboring voxels. Regional homogeneity (ReHo) is defined as the correlation of a voxel's timeseries with that of its local neighboring voxels. Therefore, the output of a ReHo analysis is a single whole brain map, in which higher values represent voxels that have strong temporal correlation with their immediate neighborhood of voxels.

The measure that is typically used to calculate ReHo is *Kendall's coefficient of concordance* (KCC). To understand this measure, consider another case where it is commonly used: to assess agreement among a group of raters. Say we ask a group of neuroscientists to rate all functional connectivity methods included in this book from their favorite to their least favorite. We can calculate KCC across all raters to determine how strongly they agree (where 1 would be perfect agreement and 0 would be no consensus at all). The advantage of KCC is that you can spatially determine the size of the neighborhood, for example, we could repeat the KCC calculation across neuroscientists located in one city, or across neuroscientists from a single lab. In the brain, KCC is used to calculate the similarity of the timecourse of voxel A to the timeseries of its neighbors within a predefined local neighborhood. Typically, the local neighborhood used in ReHo only includes the nearest neighbors (i.e., 6, 18, or 26 voxels surrounding voxel A). Once KCC is calculated for each voxel based on its neighborhood the resulting subject-wise maps can be entered into a group-level analysis (Section 4.6).

Given that ReHo is a measure of local functional connectivity, it is important to realize the potential differences between applying ReHo in three dimensional volumetric (voxel) space or on the two-dimensional cortical surface. As the surface space provides a better representation of the neural neighborhood across the heavily folded cortex, it is generally preferable to perform ReHo on the surface rather than in volumetric space.

### 4.5.1 Advantages and disadvantages of ReHo

Looking at the homogeneity of local functional connectivity is yet another way to analyze resting state functional connectivity data. ReHo aims to investigate a fundamentally different aspect of functional connectivity compared with the methods described above and, therefore, aims to add a further potentially interesting marker. However, one of the disadvantages of ReHo is that it is highly sensitive to the amount of spatial smoothing (because it is entirely driven by the local neighborhood). It is also likely to be heavily confounded by non-neuronal localized fluctuations. Additionally, ReHo is not sensitive to potential differences in the shape of the local neighborhood that is considered. This may be an important disadvantage, because it is known that the size and shape of functional regions in the brain is not uniform (for example, the cingulate cortex is elongated, while other regions such as the amygdala are smaller and more spherical). As such, it is difficult to interpret ReHo in light of other longer distance functional connectivity approaches such as SCA, ICA, and node-based measures discussed in the next chapter.

## 4.6 Group-level analysis for voxel-based methods

All of the voxel-based methods discussed in this chapter result in one or more whole-brain maps for each subject. Regardless of what this map represents (i.e., no matter if it is a ReHo or a single subject map obtained from dual regression), the main interest of any fMRI study is almost always to compare the map across subjects. To do this, it is necessary to perform a group-level analysis. At the group level it is common to compare maps across two or more different groups of subjects, or to relate the maps to non-imaging measures that vary continuously across subjects (such as performance scores, self-report measures, or symptom scores). Group-level analyses of voxel-based maps most commonly adopt the univariate *general linear model (GLM)* framework.

As described in the "General Statistics Box: Multiple Linear Regression Analysis (with the GLM)" at the end of chapter 3, the GLM is a method that is capable of general linear regression using multiple regressors, and it can be used to relate a dependent variable to one or more independent variables. In our case, the dependent variable contains all values (across subjects) from a single voxel in the subjects' voxel-based maps as obtained from any of the methods described in this chapter. This analysis is repeated separately for each voxel, which is why it is known as a *mass univariate* approach. However, performing a large number of statistical tests does result in a well-known problem of *multiple comparisons*, which is discussed in the "General Statistics Box: Multiple Comparisons Correction" at the end of this chapter. To address this multiple comparisons problem, a correction needs to be applied to the *p*-values to ensure that the statistics are valid.

The independent variables in a group-level GLM consist of one or more regressors, each with a single value per subject. These group-level regressors are defined by the researcher and they are often used to group together the subjects in the study into experimental groups. For example, a regressor with "1" for patients and "0" for healthy controls can be used to encode which subjects belong to the patient group. Regressors can also contain continuous variables, which may reflect any measure of interest, such as symptom severity or intelligence (typically entered after subtracting the mean across the group). Regressors that contain potential confounds (measures that are not of direct interest, but that should be "controlled for" in the results) can also be entered. Common examples of group-level confound regressors include age, sex, a summary score of head motion, and intracranial volume. Once the regressors have been defined, the GLM can be used to perform common tests, including paired and unpaired *t*-tests, ANOVA and regression against continuous measures, by defining *contrasts*. More information on the GLM can be found on the primer website (Short Introduction to the General Linear Model for Neuroimaging), and we strongly recommend that you read this material if you are new to the GLM.

The result of a group-level analysis using the univariate GLM framework is a whole brain map in which the value in each voxel represents either the test statistic or the *p*-value obtained from the GLM performed at each voxel. This map can be used to determine the spatial location of significant results, and answer the types of questions outlined at the start of this section.

While the GLM is by far the most common approach for group-level comparisons, other methods are available. For example, *classification methods* can be used to predict or classify an individual subject (for example, to predict whether a subject is a healthy control or a patient), based on subject functional connectivity maps. These methods are typically *multivariate* (i.e., they consider the information from all voxels at the same time, instead of testing each voxel separately). Additionally, these methods typically require that the subjects are split up into a *training dataset* (used to learn the pattern that best predicts which group a subject belong to), and a *test dataset* (used to calculate how accurately subjects can be correctly classified using the pattern obtained from the training dataset).

When performing any type of group-level analysis it is often the case that it is not possible to use parametric statistics (see "General Statistics Box" at the end of this chapter). The reason for this is that subject maps obtained from voxel-based functional connectivity measures often do not comply with the assumptions that have to be made in order to use parametric statistics. Therefore, permutation testing is recommended in order to obtain *p*-values from the group-level GLM. Permutation testing is explained in more detail in the "General Statistics Box" at the end of this chapter.

In summary, all of the voxel-based measures described in this chapter result in one or more maps per subject. These maps can be compared across subjects in a group-level analysis to identify statistically significant brain regions for the comparison of interest. Group-level analyses result in a whole-brain map of statistical results, and these then need to be interpreted in light of the localization of the finding and the research question. A discussion about the interpretation of functional connectivity findings is included in Chapter 6.

## General statistics box: Multiple comparisons correction

A common statistical problem in neuroimaging studies (that occurs in relation to null hypothesis testing) is the multiple comparisons problem (also called the multiple testing problem). In order to localize the effects of our analyses in the brain, we typically perform many tests at different locations in the brain (e.g., at each voxel). If the tests are being performed independently (like in the SCA approach described at the start of this chapter) then this is typically referred to as a *mass univariate analysis*. In standard statistics, a $p$-value threshold of 0.05 implies that we accept a 5% chance of obtaining a false result when there is no signal. Hence, on average 1 in 20 of the tests we perform will show a significant result by chance, when there was actually no real effect there. When using a $p$-value threshold of 0.05 in a whole brain analysis across 20,000 voxels (i.e., we are performing 20,000 univariate tests), 5% of those, i.e., 1000 voxels in the brain will show up as being significant when there is no true effect in those voxels (they are *false positives*). From this example it should be clear that when we perform a large number of tests it is essential to apply some form of correction to control the number of false positives and address the multiple comparisons problem. Without appropriate correction for multiple comparisons the results of a study are highly problematic and uninterpretable because it is impossible to know which findings reflect true activation/connectivity, and which are false positives. While some studies containing uncorrected results can be found in the literature, this is poor practice that is no longer accepted by journals and reviewers. When writing up your results for publication, it is essential to specify the type of correction applied, to enable replication and to help your audience interpret the findings.

In practice, the two most common approaches to multiple comparisons correction applied in neuroimaging are the *family-wise error rate correction* (FWE) and the *false discovery rate correction* (FDR). These two approaches are briefly explained here, but much more detailed information about multiple comparison correction can be found elsewhere.

### Family-wise Error rate correction

One approach to multiple comparisons correction is to consider that we have a family of tests, and we want to set a $p$-value to threshold the entire family of tests, instead of just one individual test. The approach of correcting across a family of tests is known as family-wise error rate correction (FWE). Generally speaking, family-wise error correction methods set a threshold so that instead of accepting that every individual test has a 5% chance of generating false-positive results (which is the case when we do not correct for multiple comparisons), we set a threshold such that we expect that in 5% of our studies there is one or more false positives somewhere in the brain, but in the other 95% of our studies there are zero false positives. So if we repeat the same whole brain analysis 20 times (i.e., on 20 different datasets, all containing no valid results), 19 of the univariate whole brain result maps would not contain any false positives, but one whole brain map would contain one or more false positives. Note that these types of statements represent what will happen on average if the experiment got repeated multiple times, but in any one study (or set of studies) it could be higher or lower than this (the real false positive rate of any individual study, using any thresholding method, is not known).

The most intuitive family-wise correction approach is to treat each test at every voxel as a completely independent test from all the others. To achieve this we apply a correction to the $p$-value threshold by dividing the desired threshold by the number of tests, which is called a *Bonferroni correction*. In the example above, the Bonferroni corrected $p$-value threshold would be 0.05/20,000, which is a very small number. As you can see from this example, corrected Bonferroni $p$-values quickly decrease to unacceptably small levels because of the large number of voxels (and, therefore, the large number of tests). Therefore, Bonferroni correction is not commonly adopted in neuroimaging. However, in fMRI images, two tests from two voxels that are next to each other in the brain are not truly two fully independent tests. Any type of brain map in neuroimaging typically has some amount of spatial smoothness, as a result of continuity within regions in the underlying neurophysiology, as well as the spatial smoothing intrinsic in the scanning process and applied during preprocessing. Therefore, the number of truly independent tests performed across our 20,000 voxels is considerably lower than the total number of voxels, so we need an alternative to Bonferroni correction which takes this into account.

Instead of using a Bonferroni correction to estimate the FWE threshold, more sophisticated methods are used that take the spatial smoothness and resulting lack of independence across voxels into account. In order to calculate the FWE threshold, we are interested in controlling the chance of generating a false positive finding relative to a *null distribution* (the distribution of results we would find if there were no true effects anywhere in the brain). One elegant solution is to focus on the maximum value (across voxels) of the test statistics. The reason is that if there is no true effect to be detected (i.e., our data truly follows the null distribution) then the *maximum test statistic* is the most likely to pass a set threshold and become a false positive. Therefore, we want to set a threshold using the null distribution of maximum test statistics such that 19 out of our 20 whole brain analyses do not show any false positives (i.e., even the voxel with the maximum result is below the threshold, in the case of a true null result). The null distribution of the maximum Z-statistic can be approximated using something called *Gaussian Random Field theory* (as long as a set of assumptions are met). A more detailed discussion of Gaussian Random Field theory is beyond the scope of this primer, but additional information on this topic is available in the neuroimaging literature and on neuroimaging-related websites. The approach is based on making relatively strong assumptions about the distribution of the statistics in cases where we assume that there is no signal. Therefore, this approach is referred to as a "*parametric* approach," given that we are using assumptions about parametric distributions. Alternatively, a popular *non-parametric* method that can also be used to apply FWE correction (and that

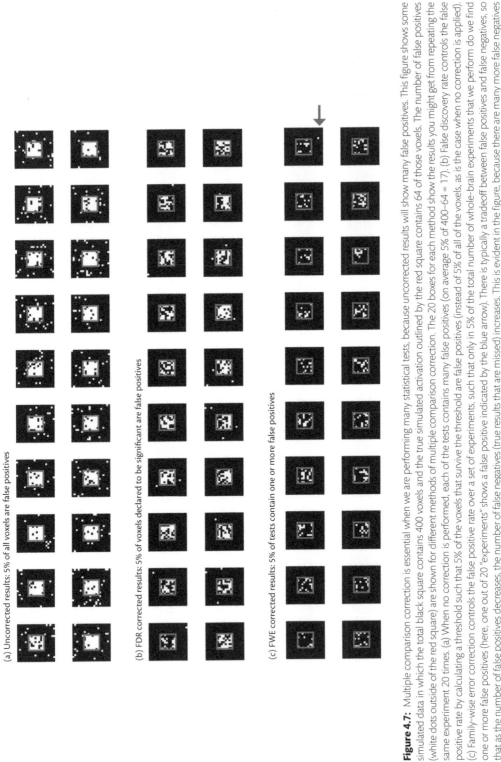

(a) Uncorrected results: 5% of all voxels are false positives

(b) FDR corrected results: 5% of voxels declared to be significant are false positives

(c) FWE corrected results: 5% of tests contain one or more false positives

**Figure 4.7:** Multiple comparison correction is essential when we are performing many statistical tests, because uncorrected results will show many false positives. This figure shows some simulated data, in which the total black square contains 400 voxels and the true simulated activation outlined by the red square contains 64 of those voxels. The number of false positives (white dots outside of the red square) are shown for different methods of multiple comparison correction. The 20 boxes for each method show the results you might get from repeating the same experiment 20 times. (a) When no correction is performed, each of the tests contains many false positives (on average 5% of 400−64 = 17). (b) False discovery rate controls the false positive rate by calculating a threshold such that 5% of the voxels that survive the threshold are false positives (instead of 5% of all of the voxels, as is the case when no correction is applied). (c) Family-wise error correction controls the false positive rate over a set of experiments, such that only in 5% of the total number of whole-brain experiments that we perform do we find one or more false positives (here, one out of 20 "experiments" shows a false positive indicated by the blue arrow). There is typically a tradeoff between false positives and false negatives, so that as the number of false positives decreases, the number of false negatives (true results that are missed) increases. This is evident in the figure, because there are many more false negatives (black voxels inside the red square) for FWE correction (c) than for FDR correction (b).

does not rely on Gaussian Random Field theory, and requires fewer assumptions) is called permutation testing, which is explained in a little more detail later on.

## False Discovery Rate correction

Another multiple comparisons correction method that you may come across is the false discovery rate (FDR). Here, instead of accepting that 5% of all voxels in the brain are false positives (as is the case without multiple comparisons correction), we decide that we are happy if 5% of the voxels declared to be significant in the brain (i.e., 1 out of 20 of the voxels that pass the threshold) are false positives. Therefore, FDR is more stringent than uncorrected results, but less stringent than FWE. The FDR threshold is calculated directly from the uncorrected $p$-values, and depends on the data. Specifically, the FDR threshold is heavily influenced by the amount and strength of the activations that are present in the whole brain map.

The crucial difference between FDR and FWE is that FDR accepts a number of false positives in every single whole-brain analysis that is performed (i.e., in each of the 20 tests using FDR in Figure 4.7 there are dots outside of the square of true activation). In fact, the number of false positives that are, on average, present after FDR correction is 1 out of every 20 active voxels that are found (when using a threshold of $p<0.05$ FDR corrected). FWE, on the other hand, controls the false positive rate more stringently, and only allows false positives in one out of every 20 whole brain analyses that are performed (so only 1 of the "tests" using FWE in Figure 4.7 shows any dots outside of the circle of true activation). Although it should be noted that, as mentioned above, the true number of false positives in any particular study is never known, regardless of the correction method that is used.

## Voxel-based versus cluster-based thresholding

For any of the correction methods described above, a corrected threshold can be calculated using a variety of different statistics. In neuroimaging, the most common statistics used to threshold a whole brain image are voxel-based and cluster-based thresholding. In voxel-based thresholding, the correction method (such as FDR or FWE) is calculated using the voxel-wise uncorrected results. Hence, voxel-based thresholding is sensitive to individual voxels in which the strength of the activation is high enough to pass a threshold.

However, in fMRI we often see activation or connectivity maps that contain spatially extended sets of voxels at any given threshold level. Cluster-based thresholding aims to use the spatial extent of the signal, and involves applying an initial, arbitrary threshold (known as the cluster-forming threshold) to the uncorrected image first and then using the size of the resulting "blobs" as input to the correction method. Hence, cluster-based thresholding uses a size-threshold to control the final false positive rate, rather than an amplitude threshold, and it is the size of the blobs that determines whether they pass the threshold. The initial cluster forming threshold that is applied to the uncorrected data is of crucial influence on cluster-based thresholding. Once you have chosen the initial threshold, the cluster size threshold is then calculated for you by the statistical method in order to set the family-wise error rate at 5%.

*Threshold-free cluster enhancement* (TFCE) is a special version of spatial statistics that aims to combine the strength of the effect in an individual voxel (i.e., the maximum test statistic used in voxel-based thresholding), with the spatial extent of the effect across voxels (i.e., the maximum number of voxels in a cluster used in cluster-based thresholding). It is, therefore, an alternative to cluster-based thresholding that does not require the (arbitrary) initial cluster forming threshold to be chosen. TFCE involves adjusting the uncorrected test statistic of each voxel in the whole brain image based on the values of the surrounding voxels, such that high voxels in large clusters are up-weighted and isolated high voxels are down-weighted. Therefore, TFCE boosts signals that are relatively weak, but that are found in a large contiguous area. Hence, this method also makes use of the fact that we expect activation or connectivity results to involve a spatial region that extends beyond a single voxel.

More detail on voxel-based and cluster-based thresholding is available in the fMRI literature. These topics are often discussed in the light of task-based studies, but essentially the same applies to group-level analysis of voxel-based resting state functional connectivity maps, because when it comes to thresholding the results of a group-level analysis it does not make a difference whether the data represent activations or connectivity.

Please note that any of the techniques introduced above for multiple comparisons correction (i.e., voxel-based and cluster-based corrections) are often applied using non-parametric statistics, and some require this (e.g., TFCE). A commonly used example of a non-parametric statistics approach (permutation testing) is discussed below.

## Multiple comparisons in more than one level of the analysis

For voxel-based methods that result in more than one map per subject (for example, for dual regression analysis performed on a set of group-ICA components) there are two levels of multiple comparisons when looking at more than one component in a group-level analysis. The conventional multiple comparisons problem across many voxels within the brain needs to be controlled (using one of the methods described above). However, when running the same group-level analysis on multiple maps (for example, on multiple group-ICA components), the results should also be corrected for the number of maps associated with independent tests that were investigated (for example, using additional Bonferroni correction). This correction is not always straightforward as not all tests will be statistically independent (for example, hierarchical testing, such as an ANOVA with follow-up post-hoc tests, does not require such corrections). While this correction for independent tests is not commonly applied in the literature to date, it is important to be aware that the risk of reporting false positives increases with the number of components maps for which you have performed the group-level comparison.

## Permutation testing

In parametric statistics it is assumed that the sample subjects are derived from a population that follows a known distribution described by a small set of parameters (mean and standard deviation). Parametric statistics are commonly adopted in neuroimaging in order to estimate test statistics and *p*-values, and most well-known statistical tests are examples of parametric statistics, including the *t*-test and ANOVA (both of which can be performed using the general linear model). While parametric statistics are easy and fast to perform, one important disadvantage is that they make several assumptions about the data. Most importantly, parametric statistics assume that the data for each population are distributed under a known parametric distribution, typically the Gaussian (Normal) distribution. However, these assumptions are often violated, for example, it is known that ICA maps do not follow the normal distribution. When the normality assumption is violated, parametric statistics become less accurate, and non-parametric methods should be considered instead.

Permutation testing forms one class of non-parametric statistics, and has gained significant popularity in neuroimaging in recent years. The advantages of permutation testing are that it makes very few assumptions about the data, and that it is extremely flexible and can be applied to any type of test statistic that can be calculated. Permutation testing is relatively easy to perform (although it can take a long time), and provides a robust and accurate estimate of the result.

The idea behind permutation testing is to use the data itself in order to build a null distribution under the assumption that the null hypothesis is true (i.e., a distribution of results that you would find if there were no underlying "true" effects). In permutation testing, this distribution of null results is created by mixing up (*permuting*) the subjects such that they do not correspond to the correct labels anymore. For example, if you are running a study to compare patients to healthy controls, then mixing up the labels would mean that both the "patient" and "healthy control" groups now contain a mixture of all subjects. Under the assumption that the null hypothesis is true (i.e., there is no difference between patients and controls in your functional connectivity measure), there essentially is only a single group and, therefore, the group-difference result should not change regardless of whether the true labels are used or whether the data are permuted. In reality, each time the labels are permuted, the result will vary a little as a result of the noise in the data. You can permute your subjects a lot of times (i.e., have many different shuffled subject orders), and after every permutation you can calculate the statistic of interest (for example, the "group difference"). After running a sufficiently large number of permutations, and each time saving the resulting value, you can combine these values into an empirical null distribution (i.e., the distribution of your test statistics under the assumption that there is no true effect in the data, and permutation becomes valid). Now you can use the un-permuted data (i.e., separate the subjects into the true patient and control groups) and calculate your real test statistic. To determine how surprising this test statistic is (i.e., to calculate a *p*-value for your real result), you can compare it to the null distribution calculated using the permuted data. For example, in order to perform a one-sided test you can divide the number of results in the empirical null distribution that were equal to, or higher than, your real result by the total number of permutations performed. This number is the *p*-value for your real result. Permutation testing can be used instead of parametric statistics, while still adopting the general linear model framework. More generically, permutation tests can be created for any test statistic, even when the associated null distribution is unknown (or cannot even be written down in closed form). The main advantage, therefore, is that we can pick a statistic that suits the needs of the investigation.

## The importance of the number of permutations

It is useful to realize that the number of permutations you perform determines the accuracy with which the $p$-value can be estimated. In order to get the most precise estimate of the $p$-value, we would have to perform all possible permutations that the data allows. However, this can often run into the millions, billions, or even more possible permutations, and it is therefore often not feasible to perform all possible permutations because it would simply take too long. For instance a simple two-sample $t$-test with 20 subjects per group has more than 137 billion possible permutations. In order to make permutation testing practical, we therefore perform a random subset of all possible permutations to get an estimate of the null distribution. However, the number of random permutations that we perform determines how accurately that distribution reflects the true distribution that we would find if we would have done all possible permutations. As a result, the number of permutations that are performed has an effect on the accuracy of the $p$-values. If we only perform 100 permutations, then we can show, via simulations, that an estimated $p$-value of 0.05 means that the true $p$-value is 0.05 ± 0.04 with 95% confidence (i.e., in 95 out of 100 times, on average, the true $p$-value will lie somewhere between 0.01 and 0.09). This makes a considerable difference when reporting a result as significant or not. There are other aspects that influence whether a result in significant or not, including the effect size and the power of the study, and therefore the number of permutations may not impact the results drastically in real studies. Nevertheless, common "safe" advice is to perform at least 5000 permutations, which would make the confidence interval 0.05 ± 0.006 (although recent work has presented various methods for speeding up the permutation inference, reducing the number of permutations needed).

The number of permutations also determines the smallest $p$-value that can be calculated. For example, when using 5000 permutations, the un-permuted value could indeed be lower than any of the permuted values. In this case the real result is right at the end of the tail of the null distribution, the $p$-value you calculate can be no lower than $1/5000 = 0.0002$. When you increase the number of permutations to 100,000, the smallest $p$-value you could now hope to find is $1/100,000 = 0.00001$. Therefore, not only does the number of permutations dictate the lowest possible $p$-value, it also sets the "granularity" of the $p$-values. Because you always divide a whole number by the total number of permutations, the steps between two $p$-values can never be smaller than one divided by the number of permutations. In the example above of 5000 permutations, the second best result is $2/5000 = 0.0004$. So, in order to be able to detect low $p$-values, and to be sensitive to small differences in $p$-values, it is also better to perform a large number of permutations.

While more permutations are typically better, there is a limit to the number of permutations that can be performed. This limit is determined by: (i) the number of subjects in your study (i.e., if you have only a few subjects, the number of ways you can shuffle them is smaller than if you have a large number of subjects), (ii) the number of permutations possible given your study design, and also by (iii) the number of shuffles that are allowed in your dataset if the observations are not independent (discussed more in the next section).

## Exchangeability

Permutation testing requires fewer assumptions than parametric statistics, but there is one fundamental assumption that needs to be met, which is known as *exchangeability*. To understand this, imagine that you are performing a twin study, in which you recruit pairs of twins where one of the twins is suffering from a disorder (for example, bipolar disorder) and the other twin has not been diagnosed with any disorders. The aim of the study is to look at the difference between the twin suffering from bipolar disorders and the healthy twin. In this case, lots of permutation options will lead to twin pairs getting broken up (i.e., one subject getting paired up with a completely unrelated subject). The difference between two unrelated subjects is likely to be much bigger than the difference between a pair of twins, and it could be due to many factors other than the diagnosis. Therefore, any permutations that lead to twin pairs getting broken up are not allowed in this scenario. The only type of permutations that fit this requirement are swaps within the twins (i.e., swapping around the healthy control twin and the twin with the diagnosis).

Generally speaking, subjects are exchangeable (i.e., can be swapped), if the permutation does not change the distribution under the null hypothesis (i.e., under the assumption that there is no signal of interest). In the example above, a permutation in which one subject would be paired with an unrelated subject would not be valid, because the null hypothesis is that there is no difference between the twins in relation to bipolar disorder. On the other hand, swapping two twins around is valid under the null hypothesis, because if there was no difference in functional connectivity related to bipolar disorder, then it does not matter whether the correct twin is labeled as the healthy control or not.

We can extend this example to a twin-study where the aim is to compare this difference between the two groups. For example, we can recruit some twin pairs where one suffers from bipolar disorder and the other is healthy, and some twin pairs where one suffers from schizophrenia and the other is healthy. The aim of the study would be to look at the difference within each twin pair, and to compare this difference between the two types of mental disorders. In this example, a further valid permutation would be to swap pairs of twins between the two groups (i.e., swapping a twin-pair from the schizophrenia group with a twin-pair from the bipolar group). For the group comparison, the null hypothesis is that there is no difference between bipolar disorder and schizophrenia in terms of difference between the twin diagnosed with one of the disorders and the healthy control twin. Therefore, a permutation that swaps a twin pair from the bipolar disorder group with a twin pair from the schizophrenia group is valid, because it would not change the distribution under the null hypothesis.

In cases where you have non-independent subjects (such as related subjects), or multiple observations for the same subject (such as a paired test of within-subject differences), it is important to account for this in the permutations. While this type of non-exchangeability adds a complication, it is usually still possible to use permutation testing by placing certain restrictions on which exchanges (permutations) are allowed.

## SUMMARY

■ Functional connectivity analysis methods can be categorized into voxel-based methods (which result in a map of functional connectivity values at every voxel in the brain) and node-based methods.

■ The following voxel based methods were discussed in this chapter:
  ▪ Seed-based correlation analysis (SCA) investigates functional connectivity between a seed region of interest and all other voxels in the brain.
  ▪ Independent component analysis (ICA) is a data-driven method that separates the data into a set of spatially independent components, where each component is described by a spatial map and an associated timecourse.
  ▪ Dual regression analysis is often used in conjunction with ICA, and aims to estimate spatial maps and timecourses that are subject-specific and can subsequently be used for statistical comparison.
  ▪ Amplitude of Low Frequency Fluctuations (ALFF) estimates the amount of low-frequency power that is present in each voxel.
  ▪ Regional Homogeneity (ReHo) estimates the amount of correlation between each voxel and the voxels that are directly neighboring it, and, therefore, aims to focus on localized, short-distance connectivity.

## FURTHER READING

■ Beckmann, C.F. (2012). Modelling with independent components. *NeuroImage, 62*(2), 891–901. Available at:. https://doi.org/10.1016/j.neuroimage.2012.02.020.
  ▪ Review paper of ICA in neuroimaging

■ Cole, D.M., Smith, S.M., & Beckmann, C.F. (2010). Advances and pitfalls in the analysis and interpretation of resting-state FMRI data. *Frontiers in Systems Neuroscience, 4*, 8. https://doi.org/10.3389/fnsys.2010.00008.
  ▪ This review paper provides summaries of many of the methods described in this chapter

■ Poldrack, R.A., Mumford, J.A., and Nichols, T.E. (2001). *Handbook of Functional MRI Data Analysis*. Cambridge University Press, Cambridge.
  ▪ While focusing on task-based research, many of the statistics (including multiple comparisons correction) are relevant to resting state functional connectivity research.

■ Zang, Y., Jiang, T., Lu, Y., He, Y., & Tian, L. (2004). Regional homogeneity approach to fMRI data analysis. *NeuroImage, 22*(1), 394–400. Available at: https://doi.org/10.1016/j.neuroimage.2003.12.030.
  ▪ Original paper on regional homogeneity

■ Zou, Q-H., Zhu, C-Z., Yang, Y., Zuo, X.-N., Long, X.-Y., Cao, Q.-J., et al. (2008). An improved approach to detection of amplitude of low-frequency fluctuation (ALFF) for resting-state fMRI: fractional ALFF. *Journal of Neuroscience Methods, 172*(1), 137–141. Available at: https://doi.org/10.1016/j.jneumeth.2008.04.012.
  ▪ Paper that introduced fALFF

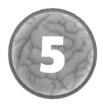

# Node-based Connectivity Analyses

The voxel-based methods introduced in Chapter 4 primarily aim at performing group-level analyses to compare the spatial organization of large-scale resting state networks. These voxel-wise approaches are powerful methods that can tell us a lot about the large-scale spatial organization of the human brain, and how this is affected in different disorders. However, these methods do not fully address how connectivity, or integration of information, is structured between distinct functional regions. Specifically, these voxel-based methods do not allow questions like: (i) how strong is the functional connection between region A and region B, or (ii) does the strength of connectivity between regions A and B differ between a group of patients and a group of healthy controls?

For these types of questions it is useful to adopt "nodes and edges" connectivity modeling. Here, "*nodes*" are different brain regions (A and B in the example above), and "*edges*" are the connections (or connection strengths) between the nodes (i.e., connection A–B). Node-based connectivity analyses are a form of graph-based connectivity modeling. A graph (Figure 5.1) is a convenient way to represent nodes and edges in a diagram.

It is important to understand the differences between voxel- and node-based resting state functional connectivity methods. The most important differences relate to the spatial scale of the methods, and what aspect of connectivity subsequent group-level comparisons are sensitive to (i.e., within-network versus between-node changes in connectivity). Voxel-based approaches typically extract relatively few extended spatial networks (generally up to a few dozen), such as the default mode network. The majority of subsequent between-subject or between-group analyses then investigate differences *within* these systems. Node-based methods, on the other hand, typically investigate connections ("edges") between a larger number of functional units ("nodes") that are spatially smaller. In node-based methods, group-level analyses compare the strength of connectivity in these edges across subjects. A node-based approach can include either a small set of nodes that only cover part of the brain (for example, the regions of a specific system of interest), or a large set of nodes covering the entire brain. It is possible, and indeed quite typical, to use voxel-based methods in order to inform subsequent node-based analyses. For example, seed-based correlation maps can be calculated for each voxel to help

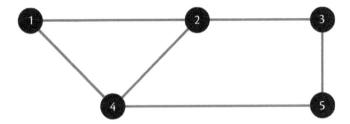

**Figure 5.1:** A graph can be used to represent connections between regions in a simple graphical format. The brain regions are displayed in black (1–5) and are called "nodes," and the connections between regions are displayed in red and are called "edges."

with node definition (see Section 5.2.3). Another example is that voxel-based methods can be used to identify regions that play a key role in a patient group of interest, and subsequent node-based approaches can study the set of identified regions in more detail.

All node-based connectivity analyses have several steps in common (see Figure 5.2); these steps are:

1. Defining the nodes, i.e., grouping voxels together into areas that are to be considered as functionally homogeneous regions.

2. Extracting the timeseries from each node. The timeseries represent the BOLD signal fluctuations over the course of the scan in each node.

3. Calculating the connectivity ("edges") between all pairs of nodes using the extracted timeseries.

4. Building a *connectivity matrix* (also called a *network matrix* or *adjacency matrix*). For example, if the node-based analysis contains 100 regions ("*nodes*" of the graph), you can build a 100 by 100 matrix that describes all possible pair-wise connections ("*edges*" of the graph). That is, the element on the 9th row and 25th column in the connectivity matrix describes the strength of functional connectivity between node 9 and node 25. A group-level node-based analysis typically has one network matrix per subject.

Each of these steps will be discussed in detail in this chapter. Various analyses that use the network matrix are discussed, although some of these further analyses may add additional steps before running between-subject/group comparisons. At the end of this chapter, we included a discussion on how to decide when to use node-based or voxel-based methods.

## 5.1  What is a node?

In order to ask questions about the connectivity between regions A and B, we first need to define these regions in terms of their precise spatial extent. It is typically not desirable to consider each voxel as a distinct "region" for multiple reasons. The first reason is because we know that the brain is organized into functional units that are larger than individual voxels, and therefore neighboring voxels often contain very similar information (i.e., the timecourses are correlated,

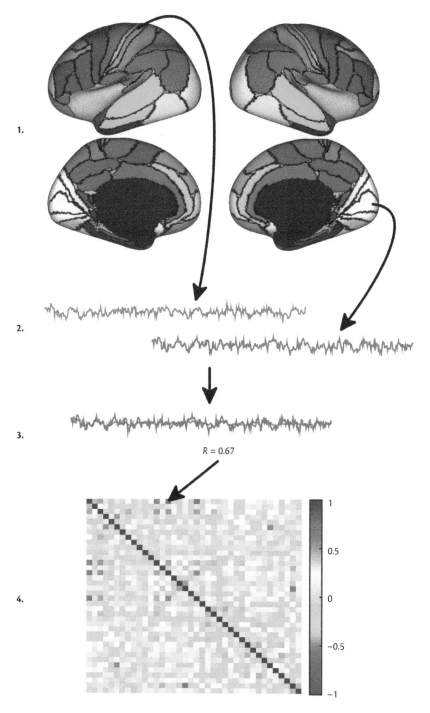

1.

2.

3.

R = 0.67

4.

**Figure 5.2:** Each node-based connectivity analysis starts with the same four steps. (1) Node definition (parcellating the brain). (2) Timeseries extraction. (3) Calculate the edge between each pair of nodes. (4) Put all edges together into a connectivity matrix.

meaning that they are partly collinear). Secondly, having fewer nodes than the large number of voxels in the brain is also beneficial because we usually have a limited number of temporal degrees of freedom (i.e., the number of time points in our resting state data is relatively small compared with the number of voxels). The temporal degrees of freedom limit the accuracy with which edges can be estimated, and puts specific limitations on the number of nodes that can be investigated for some methods of edge estimation. The issues associated with the temporal degrees of freedom are discussed at multiple points in this chapter. Finally, using all voxels as nodes would often be extremely computationally expensive; that is, estimating the edges would require a lot of computing time and memory.

From the last paragraph, it is clear that grouping multiple voxels into regions is beneficial. However, large-scale resting state networks (such as those discussed in Chapter 4) are usually too extensive to be the optimal choice for nodes. The reason for this is that, while these large-scale networks can be identified robustly from resting state data, studies of brain function suggest that sub-regions in these networks can and do act distinctly. Therefore, it is often of interest to break down large-scale networks into smaller parts, and to investigate interactions between regions in more detail. The DMN, for example, is made up of multiple regions that are known from task-based fMRI studies to be functionally distinct, including the posterior cingulate and the medial prefrontal cortex. What is useful for a node-based analysis is to separate (or "*parcellate*") the brain into functional regions that are bigger than a single voxel, yet smaller than a "network." These functional regions are also commonly called nodes, parcels, vertices, or regions of interest (ROIs). Therefore, node-based methods shift the emphasis away from large-scale spatial networks, towards a finer parcellation of the brain into smaller "functional regions." Of course, the concept of a functional node itself is somewhat simplistic, as it assumes that these functional regions are totally homogeneous with a parcel, yet distinct between parcels ("piecewise constant connectivity"). Such a simplified summary of connectivity is not a fully accurate representation of the underlying complex hierarchical organization of the brain, but is nevertheless a useful model for studying it at a certain scale.

A parcellation of the brain into nodes has multiple characteristics. First, a parcellation may be chosen to create nodes that are constrained to be spatially contiguous, or that are allowed to be distributed and contain non-contiguous sets of voxels. A *contiguous* node is a single cluster (i.e., a set of interconnected neighboring voxels), while non-contiguous nodes can contain spatially distributed, separate clusters (similar to networks, but spatially smaller). Contiguous parcels are perhaps a more intuitive version of nodes than non-contiguous parcels. However, nodes that are bilateral (and, therefore, non-contiguous) may be more biologically grounded, given that the majority of cortical regions have functional homologues in both hemispheres. Secondly, nodes can either be non-overlapping (such that no voxel is part of more than one node, which is considered a *hard parcellation*), or they can have overlapping weights for all voxels, meaning that a voxel can contribute partially to two or more nodes (a *soft parcellation*). While a hard parcellation has benefits in terms of interpretability, a soft parcellation is possibly more truthful to the underlying biology, particularly given that many regions of the brain have multiple modes of organization within the same regions. Multiple modes of organization are, for example, known to exist in the visual cortices. In primary visual cortex, the same voxels exhibit one mode of organization that represents distance of the visual stimulus from the fixation point, while a different mode of organization can be found in the same voxels when looking at sensitivity to the orientation of visual stimuli. Such complex organization likely occurs across all of the gray matter. Finally, some parcellation approaches may only include voxels in a small region of the brain (instead of parcellating the whole brain into nodes). For example, previous work has used parcellation approaches to identify sub-regions of the cingulate cortex and of subcortical structures, such as the thalamus and striatum.

From this discussion, it is clear that we do not yet understand the optimal characteristics of a brain parcellation, and it is not surprising that this is still a heavily studied research topic. There are a large number of methods available for parcellation, and several of these will be covered in Section 5.2 on "node definition." However, the "best" method is still very much up for debate and depends on your specific research question and the "scale" that you are interested in.

One complication is that it is challenging to validate a parcellation derived using resting state functional connectivity data. In some cases, such validation can be achieved using, for example, task activation data, diffusion MRI data, and/or histology (i.e., changes in microarchitecture). If the boundaries between parcels estimated using resting state data match those that can be found based on task fMRI or structural markers, this increases our confidence in the accuracy of these boundaries. These validation approaches are helpful for sensory areas, because we have good mapping methods (such as retinotopic and tonotopic mapping) for probing the different modes of organization in (early) sensory areas. However, in multimodal association cortex these functional and structural markers are more difficult to obtain, because we do not yet fully understand how information is processed in these areas. Therefore, it is significantly more challenging to find principled ways to validate parcellations in more cognitive regions.

## 5.2  Node definition

It is important to realize that node-based methods are only as good as the nodes that are fed into them, because the nodes are spatially fixed at the start of the analysis. If the functional boundary between two nodes is not placed correctly, the result is that multiple timeseries that characterize different functional regions may become mixed together (rather than averaging within a functional region, as intended). Therefore, the timeseries extracted from a node with poorly defined boundaries represents the combined signal across multiple functional areas, instead of uniquely reflecting brain function within a clearly defined and distinct area. If the timeseries extracted from one node represents a mixture of two functional regions instead of the timeseries of a single functional region, it is easy to see how the edges calculated based on such mixed timeseries are meaningless. In fact, evaluations using simulated networks have demonstrated that even a small amount of such "mixing" significantly affects all methods used for edge estimation, resulting in a severe drop in accuracy for identifying the correct system of edges from the data. This problem with boundary definition could be seen as an argument for using finer-grained node definitions, for example, using single voxels as nodes (at the extreme end). However, as discussed at various points in this chapter, there are also drawbacks of using finer-grained nodes, because including a larger number of nodes is costly in terms of temporal degrees of freedom, and may introduce problems with (near) collinearity (i.e., redundant information between node timeseries). Additionally, having smaller nodes often exacerbates problems of accurate alignment of the parcellation with individual subjects' data.

Approaches to node definition can be broadly split into atlas-based and data-driven node definition. Atlas-based nodes are available in the literature, and are typically obtained from previous studies using anatomical data ("*anatomical atlases,*" such as Harvard-Oxford, Talairach, Automated Anatomical Labeling, or Juelich), or functional MRI data ("*functional atlases,*" see Further reading for examples). Data-driven node definition, on the other hand, defines the parcellation and the boundaries of the nodes based on the same dataset that is used for subsequent node-based analyses. While atlas-based methods are derived from anatomical or functional MRI data, they are not considered here as data-driven node definition approaches because they are based on a dataset that is independent of the data used in the subsequent node-based analyses.

Given the importance of accurate functional boundaries, it is generally not advisable to use atlas-based nodes (particularly anatomical atlases). Nodes defined based on anatomical atlases are unlikely to reflect functional boundaries accurately because: (i) the methods used to derive them are often outdated; (ii) they are often based on a small sample; and (iii) different functions could be located in anatomically homogeneous regions (this is particularly likely in regions of association cortex). As such, it is advisable to use a data-driven parcellation, because it is more likely to accurately reflect functional regions in the same dataset that is used for subsequent node-based analyses.

Data-driven node definition methods aim to group voxels together into functionally homogenous regions, based on the BOLD timeseries of each of the voxels. The three main categories of data-driven parcellation methods are: (i) voxel clustering methods, (ii) linear decomposition methods and (iii) edge detection (gradient) methods. Below, each category will be briefly explained, and advantages and disadvantages will be highlighted.

Before discussing data-driven parcellation methods further, we will briefly note the importance of the number of nodes used to parcellate the whole brain (often referred to as the *dimensionality* or *model order*). For most of the methods described below, the dimensionality is a variable that is set by the researcher and is therefore somewhat arbitrary. However, it is important to appreciate that we currently simply do not have tight knowledge regarding the optimal dimensionality for parcellating the brain. In fact, multiple valid solutions are likely to exist that accurately characterize the neurobiological organization from large-scale systems to functionally specialized smaller regions. Pragmatically, the maximum dimensionality that one can expect to robustly derive from the data will be limited by the number of time points in the fMRI scan. Specifically, one can expect to robustly identify more fine-grained parcels when longer timeseries have been acquired, because longer timeseries allow for a finer-grained description of the differences in the temporal dynamics (and, therefore, enables differentiation between more functionally distinct regions). With this in mind, the next sections discuss common categories of data-driven parcellation approaches (clustering, linear decomposition, and edge detection methods).

## 5.2.1  Clustering methods for node definition

Clustering methods are popular because they offer the simplest way of grouping voxels into functionally homogeneous parcels. The general idea behind all clustering methods is to group voxels together such that the voxels in one node or parcel are more similar to each other than they are to voxels in a different node. Clustering methods commonly used in the parcellation of resting state data include k-means (centroid clustering), Ward (hierarchical clustering), and normalized cuts (spectral clustering). These clustering methods differ in the approach they use for determining which voxels are most similar to each other. For example, the K-means approach calculates the mean (called center or centroid) of each cluster, and then assigns each voxel to the most similar ("nearest") cluster center.

## 5.2.2 Decomposition methods (ICA) for node definition

*Linear decomposition* methods are an alternative to clustering for node definition, and ICA is a commonly used approach. Unlike most voxel clustering methods, approaches such as ICA do not take spatial neighborhood information into consideration (i.e., they do not differentiate between voxels that are spatially close or distant; therefore, these methods typically result in non-contiguous parcellations). In a nutshell, ICA aims to separate the data into a set of components, which are described by spatial maps that are spatially independent of each other, and associated timeseries that describe the temporal evolution of these component maps (more detail on this method is in Chapter 4). ICA provides a soft parcellation with weights for each voxel in each component that reflect how much that voxel contributes to the components. Additionally, ICA tends to produce components or nodes that are non-contiguous (for example, many ICA nodes contain bilateral functionally homologous regions).

It might be surprising to find ICA in this chapter on node-based methods, given that it was also covered in the previous chapter on voxel-based methods. However, node-definition is performed prior to node-based analyses and the node-definition actually works at the voxel level. The difference between using ICA at the large-scale network level and using ICA for the purposes of node-definition is the dimensionality of the decomposition. That is, a smaller number of components provides large-scale networks, and a large number of components results in spatially smaller nodes.

The number of components that is extracted from a group-ICA can be estimated from the data, but is also often chosen by the researcher. When comparing the results of a group-ICA analysis on the same data between a dimensionality of 25 and 100, it is clear from the component maps that many of the large-scale networks in the 25-dimensionality ICA end up being split into multiple, spatially smaller, components in the 100-dimensionality results. This implicit hierarchical nature is not an inherent feature of the analysis (as it is in Ward clustering), but instead occurs as a result of the structure present in the data. Hence, while the most commonly used dimensionalities range from approximately 10–25 for the voxel-based analyses (see Chapter 4), defining nodes using ICA is typically done using a dimensionality between 50 and 300 (depending on the number of time points available for each subject). The optimal dimensionality for either large-scale or node-based components is not known, and can probably not even be defined, given the highly complex hierarchical structure of functional regions in the brain. Therefore, deciding on an appropriate dimensionality depends on the question and hypotheses of the specific study. It can be useful to create parcellations at multiple dimensionalities and inspect the nodes visually to see how well the components separate the regions that are important for the research question. However, this should always be done prior to running the remainder of the node-based analysis, as the decision should be based on the hypothesis and research question, and not on the results!

### 5.2.3 Gradient-based methods for node definition

Both clustering and linear decomposition methods for node definition aim to group voxels together based on the similarity of their BOLD timeseries in order to create nodes. An alternative is to use the whole-brain, "seed-based" functional connectivity maps of each voxel in order to create nodes. It has been shown that there are often relatively sharp transitions in whole-brain functional connectivity patterns from one functional region to another. These sharp transitions can be used to find boundaries of the nodes using a boundary detection algorithm. Boundary detection uses the spatial gradient of connectivity (the first derivative over space, i.e., the difference from one voxel to the next) in order to find boundaries between nodes. Hence, such methods explicitly aim at identifying boundaries using changes in whole-brain functional connectivity patterns, instead of grouping voxels together based on the similarity of their timecourses (i.e., starting by finding parcels' boundaries as opposed to their centers). Note that these gradients are not only useful as a means to define nodes, but can also explain interesting variability across subjects in their own right.

### 5.2.4 Group-based versus subject-based node definition

Most data-driven methods for node definition described above are applied at the group level (i.e., they define the parcellation using data from multiple subjects). The main reasons for this are: (i) to avoid the correspondence problem (i.e., to make sure that the nodes match across different subjects), and (ii) to provide the best (most reliable) results by using as much data as possible for the parcellation. However, when nodes are defined at the group level in standard space, there is a further risk for incorrectly defined node boundaries resulting from misalignment of individual subject data to standard space. Misalignment has the potential to drive the results of a study, because, for example, registration may be more problematic in patients compared with healthy controls. Therefore, it is important to optimize registration as much as possible as discussed in Chapter 3 and in the *Introduction to Neuroimaging Analysis* primer in this series.

It may be preferable to define node boundaries at the single subject level and a lot of research is currently taking place to achieve this. However, if nodes are determined purely at the subject level, it is difficult to ensure correspondence between subjects (i.e., how we can make sure we are comparing the same functional region in subject 1 to the same region in subject 2), which is equally problematic, given that we typically aim to study groups of subjects. A preferable alternative is to define the nodes at the group level, but to include a step to refine the node boundaries in a way that is optimized for each individual subject, so that we can achieve correspondence while still allowing some flexibility in specific node boundaries (an example method that adopts this approach is to extract Probabilistic Functional Modes, see Further reading).

A related challenge is seen in node definition when the aim is to compare node functional connectivity between patients and healthy controls. When a data-driven node definition method is applied at the group level (i.e., including both patients and controls), all methods described above would be sensitive to confounds that may systematically vary across the groups (such as movement, because patients often move more than controls). In this situation, it is tempting to use only the healthy control subjects in order to define the nodes. However, this results in the nodes being biased towards the controls (i.e., being a better fit for the controls), which introduces a bias that confounds subsequent statistical comparisons between groups (as also discussed in Chapter 4). A potential alternative is to use a group of independent healthy control subjects (from a different study, which are not included in later analyses) for node definition, or indeed to use an existing functional atlas (see Section 4.3.2 for a more detailed discussion of different options). It is hopefully clear from the discussion in this section that the optimal approach to node definition is the topic of ongoing research efforts.

As a final discussion point in relation to node definition, each of the approaches for defining nodes and parcellating the brain defined above can be applied either to a volumetric or a surface-based representation of the brain (see Chapter 3). Whether it is desirable to use volumetric or surface-based representations for node-definition will depend largely on the node-definition method and also on the regions that are of interest (i.e., cortical only or including subcortical regions). Given that a large proportion of communication in the brain involves pathways between cortical and subcortical regions, only considering a surface-based cortical parcellation is unlikely to provide a complete understanding of brain connectomics. Therefore, the hybrid representation developed as part of the Human Connectome Project (using a "grayordinate" representation that involves surface-based representation of cortex and volumetric representation of subcortex and cerebellum) can be useful.

---

*Example box:* **Examples of node parcellations**

On the primer website you will find a few different parcellations that were obtained with different data-driven methods. The examples include some hard and soft parcellations, and some parcellations that are contiguous and some that are not contiguous. The examples also include ICA decompositions at different dimensionalities, to give an idea of how the set dimensionality interacts with the structure that is inherently present in the data. The aim of this is to familiarize yourself with the similarities and differences between different parcellations.

---

# 5.3 Timecourse extraction

Once the nodes have been defined, the next step in a node-based analysis is to extract a representative timecourse from each subject's resting state dataset for each node. It is important that the timecourse represents the temporal dynamics of the functional region well, as it forms the basis for calculating the edges (connectivity) between nodes.

There are two commonly used approaches for extracting the timeseries from each node. The first, and most straightforward, way to extract node timeseries is to average the BOLD data over all voxels that make up the node. The mean timeseries approach is easy to implement and is, therefore, commonly used. However, one disadvantage of the mean timeseries is that it is sensitive to potential noisy voxels in the node.

The second approach to timecourse extraction is to use dual regression (specifically, the output of the first stage; please see Chapter 4 for a more detailed explanation of dual regression). This method is commonly used when the nodes are defined using high dimensional ICA. The first step of dual regression uses the full set of group-ICA spatial maps in a multiple spatial regression, which is fit to the resting state data from each subject. Dual regression can be understood in part as a weighted average (where voxels that contribute less to the nodes are down-weighted). Importantly, dual regression is performed as a multiple regression (see detailed discussion in the "General Statistics Box: Multiple Linear Regression Analysis (with the GLM)" at the end of Chapter 3), in which all the node maps are entered into the multiple regression model simultaneously. Therefore, dual regression deals with spatial overlap between nodes by partitioning the variance between the timecourses of the components depending on their degree of correlation (i.e., taking all other spatial nodes into account). For this reason, it is valuable to enter all group-ICA spatial maps into the dual regression, including spatial maps that are considered to be noise or that are not of interest to the rest of the analysis.

In a perfect dataset that contains no noise and has perfectly defined, non-overlapping node boundaries, these two methods will result in very similar node timeseries. However, given that resting state fMRI data is very noisy, it may be preferable to use the dual regression approach (particularly when working with soft-parcellations like an ICA decomposition) in order to reduce the impact of noise. It is useful to realize that all methods essentially generate a timecourse based on some form of averaging of the voxel timecourses within the node. As a result, larger nodes that contain more voxels will undergo more averaging and, therefore, should be expected to result in smoother timecourses with less high-frequency power than smaller nodes.

## 5.4  Edge definition

Once a set of timeseries (one for each node) has been extracted for each subject, the next step in a node-based analysis is to calculate the *connectivity* between every possible pair of nodes (i.e., defining the edges). The type of information reflected by the edge can take on three different forms, namely: (i) the existence of a connection, (ii) the strength of a connection, or (iii) the direction of information flow of the connection. The edges between all possible pairs of nodes can be combined into a square matrix (in which the number of rows and columns both equal the number of nodes), which is called a network matrix (Figure 5.2).

Edges that reflect the existence of a connection are simply *binary* (0 or 1) and represent whether a functional connection between the pair of regions exists (1) or does not exist (0). However, because some pairs of brain regions may be weakly connected and others may be strongly connected, it is generally more informative to have edges that describe the strength of functional connectivity between the pair of regions (for example ranging between −1 and +1, where –1 indicates perfect anti-correlation and +1 means the timeseries are identical). Finally, it is possible to have two edges that reflect the causal flow of information from region A to region B and inversely from region B to region A. This would result in a network matrix that is not symmetric across the diagonal (because the A->B strength would not necessarily be the same as the B->A strength). Some causal connectivity measures are briefly mentioned at the end of this section, and causality is discussed in more detail in Chapter 6.

Once the edges between all pairs of nodes have been estimated (whether they reflect binary, strength, or directional edges), the resulting network matrix (i.e., the node by node matrix of all edges, one matrix per subject) is the starting point for node-based analyses at the group level.

Remember that functional connectivity is typically defined as the observed temporal correlation (or other statistical dependencies) between two measurements from different parts of the brain (as explained in Chapter 1). Therefore, the edge should reflect the relationship between two nodes (i.e., how similar the timecourses of the nodes are to each other).

## 5.4.1  Full correlation

The simplest way to estimate the similarity between two BOLD timeseries is to calculate the Pearson's correlation coefficient (i.e., the covariance between two timeseries divided by the product of the standard deviations of each of the two timeseries). This approach is also often called "full correlation" to differentiate it from partial correlation (which is described below). The advantage of full correlation is that it is easy and fast to compute and intuitive to interpret. However, the main disadvantage of full correlation is that it is sensitive to both direct and indirect functional connections in the brain. To understand the difference between direct and indirect connections, imagine a true neural system in which region A is connected to region B, and region B in turn is connected to region C (Figure 5.3). In this case, there are direct connections between A and B, and between B and C, and hence, there is only an indirect connection between A and C (via B). In this example, full correlation will show a positive connection between all combinations of regions A, B, and C without being able to distinguish between the direct and indirect connections. Hence, full correlation will show a "connection" between regions A and C (Figure 5.3). Another disadvantage of full correlation (compared with partial correlation), is that it is more sensitive to any noise confounds that are shared between multiple node timeseries and that have not been removed during preprocessing.

## 5.4.2  Partial correlation

Partial correlation is an alternative to full correlation that aims to be only sensitive to direct connections and not indirect connections. This is achieved by regressing the timeseries from region B out of the timeseries of both regions A and C before calculating the correlation between A and C. If regions A and C are only indirectly connected via B, this will remove the parts of the data in the timecourses of regions A and C that are similar, and will therefore result in a correlation that is close to zero. However, if there is still a correlation between A and C after regressing out B, then a direct connection between A and C is likely to exist. When considering a larger network, it is necessary to regress out all other node timeseries in order to calculate the partial correlation.

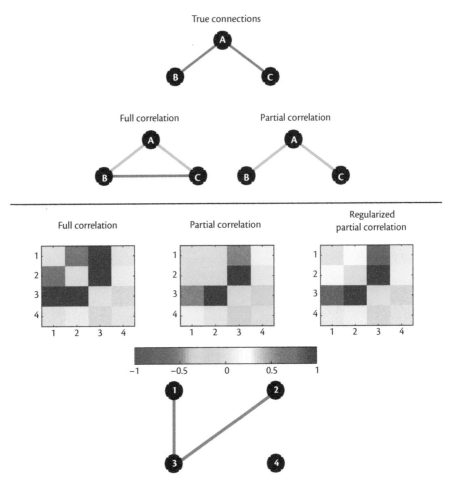

**Figure 5.3:** The difference between full and partial correlation. (Top) Full correlation identifies a connection between regions A and C, even though no direct connection exists. (Bottom) Partial correlation is only sensitive to direct connections. Therefore, in this 4-node example, the indirect connection between nodes 1 and 2 can be explained by their joined connection with node 3, and disappears when looking at partial correlation. Regularization can be used in partial correlation to reduce noisy edge estimates (compare, for example, the edge between regions 3 and 4, between partial and regularized partial correlation in the bottom part of the figure).

The advantage of partial correlation compared with full correlation is clearly that it is primarily sensitive to direct connections. However, there are two important drawbacks when using partial correlation. The first is that regressing out all other nodes before calculating an edge results in a reduction in the temporal degrees of freedom. As a result, there is a limit to the number of nodes that are possible to include in a partial correlation analysis, particularly when the resting state scan contains relatively few volumes (i.e., the timeseries are short). A second potential issue with partial correlation occurs when we have accidentally oversplit a brain region into two separate nodes, which should really be a single node. If, for example, node C from the example in Figure 5.3 is separated into C1 and C2, this will effectively remove the connection between region A and either C1 or C2 because C1 will be regressed out when looking at C2 and vice versa. So, while full correlation analysis can suffer from detecting too many connections (i.e., not distinguishing between direct and indirect connections and thereby generating "false positives"), one potential drawback of partial correlation is that it may result in *false negatives* (i.e., failing to identify connections that do exist) if we are *oversplitting* our regions into multiple nodes (given that the true nodes are often unknown, this may not be uncommon). This is a reason why having collinear nodes (or, in the extreme case, using individual voxel as nodes) is problematic.

Mathematically, partial correlation edges for a set of nodes can be estimated via calculating the inverse covariance matrix, rather than regressing out all other nodes before estimating each edge. Compared with full correlation, partial correlation edge estimation can have the effect of amplifying noise, which can be a problem when using already noisy fMRI data (particularly with short scans containing few time points). To address this noise problem, a common approach is to apply some regularization when calculating the partial correlation matrix. "Regularization" simply means that additional information is used in order to get a less noisy estimate. One regularization approach is to assume that the final partial correlation matrix should be sparse, meaning that we expect that not all of the nodes are connected to all of the other nodes and that a large number of the edges should be zero. Here, *regularized partial correlations* can be calculated, in which edges that are estimated as being close to zero are penalized and forced to become zero. Therefore, regularization results in a less noisy partial correlation matrix (Figure 5.3). It is typically a good idea to use some regularization when calculating partial correlation because resting state fMRI data are usually acquired over a relatively short period of time and are noisy. More regularization is required for shorter timeseries and/or when including more nodes, and less regularization for longer timeseries and/or when including fewer nodes (because of the degrees of freedom issue discussed previously).

Both full and partial correlation range from −1 (indicating perfect negative correlation, or anticorrelation) to +1 (perfect positive correlation). Before performing group level statistics on the edges, the correlation coefficients are often transformed to Z-statistics using Fisher's r-to-Z transformation, as in many cases this improves the statistical sensitivity and validity of later calculations.

## 5.4.3 Further options for edge definition

Many other methods for estimating connectivity are available, and examples that are used in the neuroimaging literature include coherence, Granger causality, Patel's conditional dependence, and Bayes nets. Briefly, *coherence* is the equivalent of correlation in the spectral (frequency) domain, meaning that the strength of coherence is not reduced if one timeseries lags behind the other, unlike with correlation. The other three methods aim at inferring the direction of functional connectivity (i.e., effective connectivity), as well as the strength of the connection. *Granger causality* attempts to identify causality by comparing time-shifted versions of node timeseries, under the assumption that if the timeseries of node B looks like an earlier version of the timeseries of node A then node A caused node B. While this idea of temporal dependence is intuitively attractive, in fMRI the timeseries are mediated by the slow and poorly understood hemodynamic response function (which is known to differ in delay in different brain regions). Therefore, it is unlikely that using temporal lag is the best approach for determining directionality in fMRI data. *Patel's pairwise conditional dependence* utilizes higher-order statistics, rather than just correlation, to determine the directionality of each edge. It does not suffer from the confounds that make Granger unsuitable, but is a quite noisy measure and not very accurate on many datasets. Finally, *Bayes nets* test the likelihood of different network configurations by making use of the concept of conditional independence (i.e., the idea that one set of edges may be statistically independent of each other given another set of edges). Bayes nets utilize the same kind of ideas that make partial correlation different from full correlation, modeling multiple nodes' timeseries simultaneously, to try to find the full pattern of connections and directionalities. While Bayes nets are a promising class of approaches, they have not been heavily validated yet for fMRI networks, and might not work very well if the set of connections is very "dense" (i.e., if most of the nodes are connected).

Multiple different methods for edge definition have previously been compared in a study using simulated data. The results of these simulations suggest that full and (regularized) partial correlation are among the most reliable methods for edge definition. Additionally, the results from these simulations show that estimating the directionality of functional connectivity is challenging when working on BOLD fMRI data, and that lag-based causal methods (that use temporal difference to determine directionality, such as Granger) are inaccurate when used on BOLD data.

## 5.5  Network modeling analysis

Once the node by node network matrix of all edges has been calculated for each subject, there are a number of options for further node-based analyses. Functional network modeling analysis (e.g., as implemented in FSLNets) keeps all the information in the network matrix (also called the "*netmat*") and performs group-level analyses on this. Hence, it uses the network matrix to ask the research questions, such as: i) which edges differ in strength between the patient and healthy control groups?, or ii) which edges vary across subjects in a way that is correlated with a continuous behavioral variable of interest (for example IQ)?.

In order to compare the network matrix across subjects in a group-level analysis, the subject network matrices are sometimes first combined into one large (number of subjects by number of edges) matrix (Figure 5.4). In the case of defining edges in terms of full or partial correlation this is done by discarding one half of the network matrix (which contains the same information as the other half, because the matrix is symmetric, i.e., mirrored across the diagonal), and then reassembling half of the node by node matrix of edges from each subject into one long row. Multiple subjects can then be stacked onto subsequent rows to form a large subjects-by-edges matrix. This matrix can be used to perform group analyses as described below.

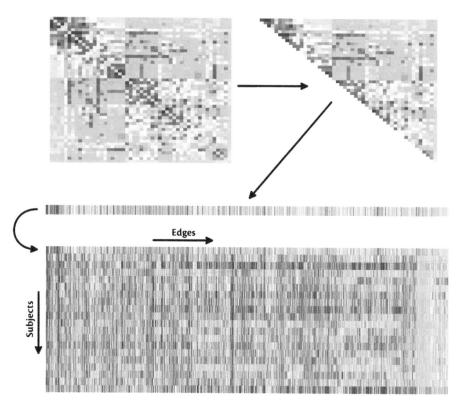

**Figure 5.4:** A network matrix from a single subject can be mapped onto one line by removing the redundant part of the symmetric matrix and unwrapping it so that all edges are next to each other. Subjects can then be stacked below each other to form a matrix ready for group-level analysis.

---

*Example box:* **Calculating subject and group network matrices**

In this example you will calculate and visualize network matrices from individual subjects, and perform a simple group analysis to estimate the group-level network matrix. On the primer website you will find a set of subject timeseries that are ready for further network modeling analysis. You will estimate the network matrix using both full and partial correlation in order to look at the similarities and differences between these edge definition approaches. The aim of this example is to familiarize yourself with the types of results obtained from a network modeling analysis.

---

## 5.5.1  Univariate group-level network analysis

There are multiple different approaches to performing a group-level network modeling analysis. The first is to use a mass univariate method, which treats each edge separately and performs the same statistical test independently at each edge. The mass univariate method typically uses the General Linear Model (GLM) in exactly the same way as in voxel-based analysis, but instead of comparing voxels, the GLM now compares edges. The GLM framework is capable of many types of comparisons, including comparing two or more groups (paired or unpaired), ANOVA, and regression against continuous variables (see the "General Statistics Box: Multiple Linear Regression Analysis (with the GLM)" in Chapter 3). When a GLM is applied separately to each edge, it is important to correct the resulting *p*-values for the number of edges you are testing to control the rate of false positive results that occur by chance when doing a large number of tests (i.e., multiple comparison correction). Permutation testing ("General Statistics Box: Multiple Comparisons Correction" in Chapter 4) is often used to obtain *p*-values of the group comparison for each edge.

## 5.5.2  Multivariate group-level network analysis

The second option for performing a group-level network modeling analysis is to perform a multivariate *classification* (or prediction) analysis, which combines information across multiple edges in order to find patterns of edges that best differentiate subjects in group 1 from subjects in group 2, for example. Classification algorithms use a set of features (in our case the edges) to find patterns of edges that best predict whether a given subject is part of group 1 or group 2 (or to predict one or more continuous variables). The most common class of classification methods are linear classifiers, such as linear discriminant analysis (LDA), but non-linear methods also exist.

There are four steps in a typical classification analysis. First, *feature selection* is often performed to reduce the number of edges that are included in the classification analysis (as a very large number of noisy edges can reduce the classifier performance). This can be achieved by thresholding the network matrix, for example only including the top 10% of edges that are either strongest overall, or that show the biggest group difference as features. Secondly, the subjects need to be split up into a training and test set of subjects. Thirdly, the training dataset (which includes information about which group the subjects belong to) is used to train the classifier. Here, the classification algorithm learns a function that maps a pattern of edges onto the subject labels. Fourthly, the classifier now has to label the test subjects based on the function it estimated from the training subjects. The main result of the analysis is the *classification accuracy*, which is the percentage of test subjects that were accurately labeled.

It is also possible (for linear multivariate methods) to look at which edges contributed to the multivariate pattern that was used for the classification (also called the classification weights). However, it is important not to overinterpret the edges that contribute most to the classifier's predictive accuracy. For example, some edges may have a weight that is close to zero in the classifier pattern even though it is, in fact, different between groups 1 and 2. This can happen because multiple edges contain the same information and in this case only one of the edges shows up in the pattern. On the other hand, it is possible that an edge receives a high predictive weight in the pattern, even though it does not contain any direct information about the difference between groups 1 and 2. For example, edges that cancel out noise that is correlated with the two subject groups would increase the accuracy of the overall pattern and, therefore, receive a high weight (i.e., the classifier would use this edge). Hence, the classification weights are not always helpful in order to interpret the most important edges for the classifier. However, some alternative methods can be used to obtain more interpretable edge coefficients (see Further reading for more information).

The advantage of a mass univariate approach, such as GLM is that it is straightforward to interpret because the result for each edge only relates to the information contained in that edge. However, the univariate method is rarely sensitive to small changes in edge strength as these would not survive the relatively harsh correction for multiple comparisons that would be required to control for the risk of finding a result by chance given the number of tests that are performed (see "General Statistics Box" at the end of Chapter 4). Multivariate techniques, on the other hand, are potentially sensitive to small changes in edge strengths (across multiple edges) because they search for a multivariate pattern. However, as a result it is more challenging to interpret the weights produced by a classification, because the resulting pattern has to be inferred as a whole (although the classification/prediction accuracy is more straightforward to interpret).

### 5.5.3  Advantages and disadvantages of network modeling analysis

The main advantage of network modeling analysis, compared with voxel-based methods such as ICA, is that it makes it possible to perform different types of functional connectivity research. Specifically, network modeling analysis enables us to look at changes in connection strength between specific regions of interest in a relatively hypothesis-driven approach compared with voxel-based methods (see Section 5.9). Additionally, node-based methods play an important role in mapping the functional connectome of the human brain. Mapping the connectome involves identifying the (functional) connectivity between all functional regions in the brain. Therefore, a network modeling analysis that builds a network matrix of edges between a comprehensive set of regions covering the whole brain is an important method for connectomics.

However, it is important to be aware of the disadvantages of network modeling analysis. The most important drawback of performing a network modeling analysis is that the nodes must be spatially defined at the start and cannot change shape or size as part of the analysis. As discussed in Section 5.2, if the spatial boundaries of nodes do not accurately reflect the underlying functional organization of the brain, this will render the results of a network modeling analysis completely uninterpretable.

## 5.6  Graph theory analysis

Graph theoretic techniques can provide further node-based analysis approaches, which also use the network matrix of edges we have calculated (which is also commonly called the "graph"). However, instead of directly comparing the network matrix across (groups of) subjects, graph theoretic approaches use it to extract higher level summary measures that describe aspects of network functioning. Typically, graph theory analysis uses correlation to calculate the network matrix edges, and subsequently thresholds the network matrix into a binary matrix (meaning that the edges are either 1 or 0, i.e., either there is or there is not an edge between any two nodes). As a result of this binarization process, typically only 10–20% of the edges with the strongest connectivity are retained. This binarized (also called "unweighted") network matrix can be used to extract local and global measures of network characteristics. The most common graph theoretic measures are described below, and shown in Figure 5.5.

*Node-wise summary measures:*

- The *minimum path length* between two nodes is defined as the smallest number of edges that are needed to travel from node A to node B.
- The *clustering coefficient* of a node measures the number of other nodes that it has edges with, which also have edges with each other. Hence, a high clustering coefficient means that if nodes A and B are both connected to node C, they are also likely to be connected to each other. Calculating the clustering coefficient takes into account the number of connected triangles of nodes.
- The *degree* of a node is defined as the number of other nodes it is connected to. Nodes with a degree that is larger than the averaged degree in the graph are called *hubs*. Hubs are often densely connected to other hubs (usually via long-distance connections) forming a so-called *"rich club"* of nodes.

*Global summary measures:*

- The local measures for minimum path length and clustering coefficient can be averaged to calculate the mean path length and clustering coefficient of the whole graph.

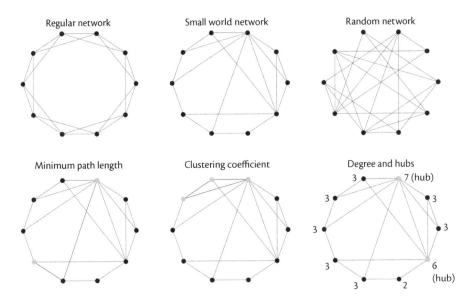

**Figure 5.5:** Graph theory analysis uses the network matrix (usually after thresholding) to calculate summary measures of network functioning. These measures relate to the organization and efficiency of the network and describe things like the minimum path length, clustering coefficient, degree, and small worldness.

Additionally, the distribution of degrees over all nodes can be informative in terms of the likelihood of any specific degree being present in the network.

■ *Global efficiency* is inversely proportional to the average minimum path length (i.e., one divided by mean path length), and is a measure of the efficiency of the graph as a whole.

■ *Small worldness* is a characteristic of networks that is found in many complex systems such as social networks, the internet, and also the brain. Small world network organization means that nodes are densely connected locally, with a few long-distance connections between hubs. Using hubs in this way is beneficial in terms of network efficiency because it means that nodes are well connected without the need for a large number of random connections. Hence, small world networks are characterized by a low minimum path length and high clustering coefficient. The small worldness of a network can be calculated by comparing the average minimum path length and average clustering coefficient of the network against a randomly connected network.

These graph theoretic summary measures can be calculated for each subject and compared between groups to inform us about differences in network organization between, for example, patients and healthy controls. Regular statistics such as a *t*-test can be used to compare the summary measures, because graph theory measures typically summarize the functional connectivity into a single value per subject. One of the advantages of graph theory is, therefore, that it does not suffer from multiple comparison problems (because the results are a single value rather than a whole brain map or network matrix per subject). Nevertheless, if multiple graph theoretic measures are being compared then these will need to be corrected for multiple comparisons. Additionally, the single value summary measure obtained from graph theory may be useful as a simple biomarker of connectivity.

## 5.6.1  Eigenvector centrality mapping (ECM)

A method closely related to degree is called eigenvector centrality mapping (ECM). ECM is really a voxel-wise method, but we are mentioning it in this chapter because it is very strongly linked to the graph theoretical measures discussed above. The aim of ECM is to identify voxels that play a central role in the network structure. It works by assigning a value to each voxel, which represents both the number of other voxels it is connected to, and also the degree of those connected voxels in turn (i.e., connections to hubs obtain a stronger weight). The result of an ECM analysis is a single map that represents how strongly each voxel is correlated with other regions that in turn play an important role in the network structure.

## 5.6.2  Advantages and disadvantages of graph theory analysis

While it is appealing to summarize complex networks into a single value per subject, there are serious potential disadvantages to this approach. First, the network matrix used for graph theory is often the full correlation matrix, which includes both direct and indirect connections between nodes (as explained earlier in this chapter), and which is more sensitive to widespread (e.g., global across the brain) confound signals. Secondly, thresholding network matrices into binary graphs removes a lot of potentially important information from the unthresholded (weighted) matrix. Finally, the further reduction of the binarized edge information into summary measures again runs the risk of removing valuable information. As a result, graph theory metrics are quite far removed from the original data, and it can be difficult to determine how to understand changes in graph theoretic summary measures in terms of brain functioning. Nonetheless, the graph theory approach will benefit from ongoing improvements in node definition, edge estimation, and use of weighted (un-thresholded) network matrices to calculate graph theoretic measures.

## 5.7  Dynamic causal modeling

Up until now, we have primarily discussed resting state fMRI methods for estimating functional connectivity. Hence, the methods covered so far are not aimed at investigating the directionality of the connection. However, often an aim is to gain an understanding of *effective connectivity*, which reflects the information flow in the underlying neural structures (for example, node A driving node B). Effective connectivity, and the relationship to underlying biology and to interpretation of findings, is discussed in more detail in Chapter 6. Note that an effective connectivity network matrix is not symmetric, because the connection strength from region A to region B is not the same as the connection strength from region B to region A. Hence, the directionality of the connection is reflected in the network matrix, making it non-symmetrical. The methods that have been covered so far are also observational approaches to resting state fMRI data, which do not explicitly attempt to model the underlying physiology. *Dynamic causal modeling* (DCM) is a node-based method that aims to build biophysically plausible models of networks at the neural level that can estimate directional edges observed in fMRI data.

DCM differs from the other node-based methods mentioned in this chapter in three important ways. First, DCMs are *generative*, meaning that they explicitly model the firing of neural populations within nodes, which are then passed through a model of the hemodynamic response function and the imaging process to predict BOLD data. An advantage of this approach is that DCM is, in theory, the method that is most strongly grounded in biology, such that the results can potentially be used to interpret the neurophysiology of the network. Secondly, DCM can estimate effective connectivity weights separately for connections in two different directions (A>B and B>A), if these are both included in the specified network model (and if the data and its dimensionality supports the inference). Thirdly, DCM is a *Bayesian* analysis, which means that parameters in the model have associated *prior beliefs* (which can use empirical knowledge to constrain the analysis), and that the result has a *posterior distribution* (which reflects the amount of uncertainty of the fitted model parameters). The DCM approach works by comparing a set of different model configurations (i.e., different ways of drawing edges between nodes), and finding the set of edges that has the best Bayesian *model evidence*.

Hence, DCM aims to find the configuration of edges that is most likely to result in the data that was actually observed.

### 5.7.1  Advantages and disadvantages of DCM

While the biological grounding of DCM is attractive (as this should arguably be an important goal of connectomics), at present, there are several limitations to using the DCM approach in order to understand resting-state connectivity. The first limitation of DCM is the same as its strength and lies in the hemodynamic model that is used to link the firing of neural populations to BOLD data. It is known that different areas of the brain differ in the amplitude, delay, and overall shape of the hemodynamic response function, and that this varies from person to person and from one day to the next. Our knowledge of this complex hemodynamic response function is quite limited, and the true complexity of the biological processes from neuronal activity to the BOLD signal may not be captured by the specific models used within DCM. This possible mismatch may result in incorrect edge strength estimates within the DCM and, therefore, potentially lead to selecting the wrong configuration of edges. The second main limitation of DCM is that it is necessary to compare different model configurations in order to find the best fit. If we are interested in the whole brain, the number of possible ways to draw edges between the nodes increases dramatically with the number of nodes included. Therefore, the number of possible models to compare (the "full model space") quickly becomes extremely large and an analysis that explores all options will take a very long time. Additionally, it is possible that multiple configurations of edges could result in the data that we are observing and it may not be possible to distinguish between them to find the correct result. The large number of nodes often used in resting-state analysis also leads to a very large number of parameters in the DCM model, which may be difficult to estimate (a challenge that is made even harder when applying DCM to resting-state data, as opposed to task-fMRI data, because the latter is able to take advantage of the known timings of the experimental paradigm). Nonetheless, it may be possible to address some of these limitations with additional research and resources. If the impact of these limitations can be reduced, DCM studies will be interpreted with greater confidence, and DCM may well be a powerful method allowing us to draw stronger conclusions about the causal interactions between different neural populations.

## 5.8  Dynamic and non-stationary methods

All of the voxel- and node-based methods described so far have implicitly assumed that networks and edges are stable over an extended period of time. However, given that the brain is likely to be cognitively active during a resting state scan (i.e., subjects are "thinking"), it is likely that connectivity strength (i.e., the edge strength between two nodes) may change over time during the course of a scan. Changes in functional connectivity over time are potentially very interesting in order to study the current mental state of a subject, or to trace functional connectivity as we engage in different cognitive processes and/or mood states over time. As a result, there is growing research that aims to investigate such connectivity dynamics.

In the literature on changes in functional connectivity over time, there are multiple different terms that are used relatively interchangeably. *"Dynamics"* is a general description of how a signal evolves over time. *"Non-stationarity,"* on the other hand, has a very precise mathematical meaning that is different from dynamics. A timeseries can be called non-stationary if there is a fundamental change over time in any one of the statistical properties, such as the mean and variance, which describe the distribution of the signal. Given this specific definition, it is relatively difficult to find evidence of non-stationary functional connectivity (because you need to model the parameters of the distribution and show a significant change in these, rather than simply observing changes in the observed samples). Therefore, it is often a good idea to refer to changes in functional connectivity over time using the more general term of "dynamics." In either case you will need to perform rigorous statistical analysis on estimates of dynamics in order to establish that these changes are not simply driven by noise (discussed more in Section 5.8.1).

## 5.8.1  Windowed analysis

A common class of approaches to studying dynamic functional connectivity is to adopt a windowed node-based analysis. For a *windowed analysis*, the timeseries are partitioned into sections (windows) and the edge strength is calculated separately for each window. For example, if a study acquired data during a 10-minute scan, and a window length of 30 seconds is used, then a series of 20 edges are calculated for each pair of nodes. Hence, instead of ending up with one node-by-node connectivity matrix per subject, we obtain 20 node-by-node connectivity matrices for each subject (one for each window of 30 seconds). In this example, each time point is only part of a single window and, therefore, the windows do not overlap. More commonly, a *sliding window* approach is used in which the window slides from one time point to the next (i.e., the first window covers 1–30 seconds, and the second window covers 2–31 seconds, etc.). There are a number of complications that arise when using a windowed analysis compared with a stationary node-based analysis of the entire timeseries, some of which require additional steps in the analysis pipeline. Four of these complications will be discussed below, and at the end of this section an alternative method (coherence) that addresses some, but not all of the complications, will be described.

The first complication of windowed analyses is noise. While the effect of noise is important to consider in any analysis on fMRI data, it is easy to understand that the edges will be considerably more sensitive to noise if they are calculated using only 30 seconds compared with using the full 10 minutes of data in our example. Therefore, it is likely that the results show fluctuations in the edge strength over time simply as a result of noise, instead of reflecting true underlying dynamic changes in the connection between the two nodes. There is a trade-off in terms of the *window length*, such that longer windows will give less noisy estimates of connectivity, but at the cost of being less sensitive to detecting the sorts of dynamic changes in edge strength that are of interest (and mixing together more distinct states that have occurred during the longer window). For this reason, studies commonly use a range of window lengths to show that the results do not change drastically as a function of window length. Typical window lengths used in resting state fMRI range from 30 to 60 seconds. The window length interacts with the TR of the data, because the number of time points in a 30-second window is 30 divided by the TR. Therefore, it is advisable to acquire data with a short TR for windowed analysis, for example using a multiband sequence (as described in Chapter 2).

Importantly, even with a short TR and a range of window lengths, noise may still have a large influence on the results, and is likely to cause some observed fluctuations in the edges. In order to interpret the observed fluctuations as evidence of dynamic changes in the underlying connection, rather than being caused by the random noise, it is vital to compare the results against fluctuations that you would observe if the data were purely driven by noise (i.e., to perform a statistical comparison). Therefore, we need to obtain a null distribution that describes the range of fluctuations that we might observe in data that does not contain any real dynamic changes in connectivity over time. There are multiple options for creating such a stationary null distribution. One option is to use the data itself and to perform a windowed analysis to calculate edges between node timeseries that are extracted from two separate subjects. Given that the node timeseries were not derived from the same brain, we would expect these "edges" to be driven by noise and any dynamic changes in connectivity over time to occur as a result of noise. Other options that you may come across in the literature are randomizing the phase of each of the timeseries, or using surrogate data that has been generated to have the same properties as the BOLD data, but are known not to contain dynamic changes. The true result can then be compared against a null distribution in order to determine whether the observed dynamics are significantly greater than what would be observed as a result of noise in data that does not contain dynamic changes.

A second complication of windowed analyses is one that is often overlooked, and it relates to the number of cycles that a signal of a particular frequency goes through within one window. As discussed in Chapter 1, the majority of the power in a BOLD signal lies in the low frequencies (roughly between 0.001 and 0.03 Hz). A signal with a frequency of 0.01 Hz takes 100 seconds to go through a full cycle. Therefore, if the length of a window is between 30 and 60 seconds, the signal may arbitrarily be in a high or in a low part of its cycle in any one window. If the windowed analysis only "sees" part of the cycle it could therefore incorrectly estimate an edge between two nodes that varies a lot, simply because of these arbitrary high and low parts that are only a short part of the same signal. Therefore, it is extremely important to high-pass filter the BOLD data prior to timeseries extraction when performing a windowed analysis. The high-pass filter will remove any slow fluctuations from the data below a certain cut-off frequency (as explained in Chapter 3). Therefore, functional connectivity estimated in a windowed analysis is driven by relatively high-frequency fluctuations, as opposed to the analyses discussed earlier in this primer, which are more strongly influenced by low-frequency fluctuations (as a result of the HRF).

The third complication of a windowed analysis relates to the amount of outputs that are generated. Instead of obtaining one network matrix per subject, a windowed analysis results in one network matrix per window per subject. It is therefore more challenging to perform statistics and also to interpret and visualize such a large number of results. One aspect that is often of interest is to identify recurring connectivity states that are present at multiple points in the resting state scan. A common approach to identify such recurring functional connectivity patterns from a windowed analysis is to group the resulting network matrices using clustering or principal component analysis (PCA). An alternative to this approach (i.e., windowed analysis followed by clustering), is to explicitly model the hidden states and their transitions (for example, using a Hidden Markov Model).

The fourth, and final, complication of windowed analysis relates to the interpretation of observed dynamics in functional connectivity. There are many different things that could drive such fluctuations in edge strength. For example, changes in edge strength of a node could mean that this node is part of two or more different networks, and is changing its connections over time as it is switching from one network to the other. Alternatively, it is possible that the node is part of the same single network, but that the strength of connections within that network fluctuate over time. Gaining a full understanding of these types of dynamics and their implications for systems neuroscience and for subject behavior, while challenging, is potentially important in order to fully map whole brain connectomics.

## 5.8.2  Time-frequency coherence methods

Time-frequency coherence methods provide an alternative to windowed methods. Coherence approaches result in a time-frequency spectrum that provides a rich view of the relationship between two timeseries, both over a range of frequencies and across the time points of the scan. *Wavelet* analysis effectively varies the window length depending on the frequency, and can therefore be understood as separating the node timeseries into multiple frequencies and picking the optimal window length to look at each frequency (i.e., longer windows for low frequencies and shorter windows for high frequencies). The way this is achieved is by first performing a wavelet transform (which is comparable to a Fourier transform, but located in time as well as in frequency) on each of the timeseries. Those time-frequency transforms of the node signals can then be used to compare two nodes to investigate coherence (i.e., do both nodes have high and correlated power in the same frequency at the same time), as well as the relative phase between the nodes (are they correlated or anticorrelated at a specific frequency and time). The coherence approach removes the need for high pass filtering that is required for windowed analysis (as the window length is optimally chosen as part of the method). However, the same complications of noise, difficulty in summarizing large sets of results, and interpretation challenges are shared between coherence and windowed methods.

In summary, there is growing interest in studying changes in functional connectivity that occur over time. If you are performing this type of research, it is important to adopt the correct terminology, by distinguishing between dynamic and non-stationary connectivity. Additionally, it is helpful to carefully consider which method is best suited for studying the types of changes over time you expect to find. One aspect to consider is the time scale over which you expect to observe the types of changes that are of interest. It is likely that changes in the cognitive state of a subject may vary relatively little, because the types of variability in behavior, mood and psychological state typically occur relatively slowly (i.e., over the course of hours or days, rather than within a 10-minute scan). One option is to experimentally induce changes in cognitive state (state-dependent resting fMRI) with the use of an experimental manipulation (this is discussed in more detail in Section 6.1.2).

## 5.9 When to use voxel-based versus node-based approaches

At this point, you should have a relatively good understanding of the different voxel-based and node-based methods that are available to study functional connectivity. An important first step in your own research in this field is to decide what method to use for your study. As we mentioned at the start of Chapter 4, there is no single right method, and all of the approaches discussed in Chapters 4 and 5 are commonly used and play a role in the overall field of functional connectivity. However, for any given study there are methods that are more or less appropriate. That is, some methods are better suited to some particular research questions.

To decide whether a voxel-based or node-based method is best for your study, a key question to ask yourself is: do you know which brain regions are likely to play a key role in your study (from your own research, or from the previous literature)? If you know that you are interested in functional connections between a specific set of regions that together form a cognitive system, then a node-based analysis may be the most suitable approach. For example, it may be of interest to investigate a set of regions known to be involved in emotion regulation, in order to determine which edges change when participants are relaxed, compared with when participants have just experienced a stressor. On the other hand, if you do not have strong prior knowledge about which brain regions are of interest, then a voxel-based method may be helpful to initially identify key regions (which may lead to subsequent investigations with node-based methods). Alternatively, you may know which large-scale networks may play a key role in your study (such as, for example, the DMN), but it might not be clear what type of change you might see in the network (i.e., whether there may be a change in the spatial configuration, or a change in connectivity strength between specific regions). In this case, voxel-based methods may be a better option to use, even though you know which regions are of interest. This is related to the fact that voxel-based and node-based methods differ in the type of output they provide. Voxel-based analyses are spatial methods that result in maps, whereas node-based analyses are temporal methods that result in a connectivity matrix instead of a map. The maps resulting from voxel-based methods can tell us something about changes in the localized strength of connectivity, as well as changes in spatial shape and size of networks. In node-based methods, on the other hand, the nodes are defined prior to the analysis and their shape and size do not change as part of the analysis. Therefore, a disadvantage of node-based methods is that they are strongly influenced by how well the overall spatial definition of the nodes matches the boundaries of functional regions in individual subjects (as discussed in Section 5.2). The result of a node-based analysis is typically either a connectivity matrix or a summary measure derived from a connectivity matrix. Therefore, node-based methods are well suited for studying differences in connectivity strength between a set of known regions, whereas voxel-based methods are preferable to localize changes within large-scale networks (which may include changes in network shape). Importantly, these two different approaches to the data can be combined, where voxel-based methods are used to validate the choice of node definition, and node-based approaches inform about the connectivity between those nodes.

## SUMMARY

- Node-based functional connectivity methods use a graph-based approach to modeling connectivity, which includes nodes (a group of voxels that together make up a functional region) and edges (the strength of connectivity between each pair of nodes).

- There are several steps that are part of each node-based functional connectivity method, namely:
  - *Node definition*: data-driven methods for brain parcellation are best; options include clustering, ICA, and gradient-based methods.
  - *Timeseries extraction*: often the mean timeseries averaged across all voxels in a node.
  - *Edge definition*: common methods include full and partial correlation (correlation after regressing out the timeseries from all other nodes).
  - *Network connectivity matrix*: entering the edge strength for each possible pair of nodes into a matrix.

- Once the network connectivity matrix is calculated, multiple further node-based analyses can be performed:
  - *Network modeling analysis* performs group-level statistics on the network connectivity matrix that was calculated for each subject.
  - *Graph theory analysis* estimates local and global summary measures after binarizing the network matrix; common summary measures include degree, global efficiency, and small worldness.
  - *Dynamic causal modeling* is a method for effective connectivity (i.e., for inferring the directionality of connections). It works by comparing different node configurations, and using a model that starts at the neural firing level to determine which of the configurations best matches the BOLD data recorded, and inferring the biophysical model parameters.
  - *Dynamic measures* aim to determine temporal changes in connectivity over time and a common method for this is to calculate a network matrix for multiple short time windows.

## FURTHER READING

- Craddock, R.C., James, G.A., Holtzheimer, P.E., 3rd, Hu, X.P., & Mayberg, H.S. (2012). A whole brain fMRI atlas generated via spatially constrained spectral clustering. *Human Brain Mapping*, *33*(8), 1914–1928. Available at: https://doi.org/10.1002/hbm.21333.
  - A commonly used parcellation.

- Eickhoff, S.B., Thirion, B., Varoquaux, G., & Bzdok, D. (2015). Connectivity-based parcellation: critique and implications. *Human Brain Mapping*. Available at: http://doi.org/10.1002/hbm.22933.
  - A critical review of parcellation methods.

- Fornito, A., Zalesky, A., & Bullmore, E. (2016). *Fundamentals of Brain Network Analysis*. Elsevier, Amsterdam.
  - Covers graph theoretical analysis of connectomes data

■ Friston, K.J. (2011). Functional and effective connectivity: a review. *Brain Connectivity*, *1*(1), 13–36. Available at: http://doi.org/10.1089/brain.2011.0008.
    ▫ A good review of the differences between functional and effective connectivity.

■ Glasser, M.F., Coalson, T.S., Robinson, E.C., Hacker, C. D., Harwell, J., Yacoub, E., et al. (2016). A multi-modal parcellation of human cerebral cortex. *Nature*, *536*, 171–178 . Available at: https://doi.org/10.1038/nature18933.
    ▫ Parcellation of the cortex based on multimodal HCP data.

■ Harrison, S.J., Woolrich, M.W., Robinson, E.C., et al. (2015). Large-scale probabilistic functional modes from resting state fMRI. *NeuroImage*, *109*, 217–231. Available at: https://doi.org/10.1016/j.neuroimage.2015.01.013.
    ▫ Paper that described Probabilistic Functional Modes (an alternative decomposition to ICA, which estimates group maps and subject maps at the same time).

■ Haufe, S., Meinecke, F., Gérgen, K., et al. (2014). On the interpretation of weight vectors of linear models in multivariate neuroimaging. *NeuroImage*, *87*, 96–110. Available at: https://doi.org/10.1016/j.neuroimage.2013.10.067.
    ▫ A discussion on the interpretation of multivariate classification methods for group level analysis.

■ Smith, S. M., Miller, K. L., Salimi-Khorshidi, G., Webster, M., Beckmann, C. F., Nichols, T. E., et al. (2011). Network modelling methods for FMRI. *NeuroImage*, *54*(2), 875–891. http://doi.org/10.1016/j.neuroimage.2010.08.063
    ▫ A paper testing the importance of accurate node definition and comparing edge definition methods with the use of simulations.

■ Thirion, B., Varoquaux, G., Dohmatob, E., & Poline, J-B. (2014). Which fMRI clustering gives good brain parcellations? *Frontiers in Neuroscience*, *8*, 167. Available at: http://doi.org/10.3389/fnins.2014.00167.
    ▫ An overview and comparison of three clustering approaches to whole brain parcellation.

■ Yeo, B.T.T., Krienen, F.M., Sepulcre, J., Sabuncu, M. R., Lashkari, D., Hollinshead, M., et al. (2011). The organization of the human cerebral cortex estimated by intrinsic functional connectivity. *Journal of Neurophysiology*, *106*(3), 1125–1165. Available at: https://doi.org/10.1152/jn.00338.2011.
    ▫ A commonly used parcellation of the cortex

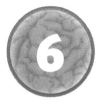

# Interpretation

An important consideration for any resting state fMRI study—irrespective of the functional connectivity method used, or the population studied—relates to the question of how the findings should be interpreted. It is extremely important to be aware of the limitations and caveats of the measured signal. When it comes to interpreting the findings of your resting state functional connectivity study, there are several important things that require careful consideration. Specifically, there are multiple factors that play an important role in determining the final analysis results, namely:

**A.** The *psychology* of the subject (the mental state and ongoing psychological processes during the scan).

**B.** The *physiology* of the BOLD signal (the characteristics of the BOLD signal and the intermediate physiological mechanisms that give rise to the signal).

**C.** The *methodology* of the analysis approach (the preprocessing and analysis pipeline choices).

To help guide the challenging process of interpretation, this chapter sets out to summarize each of these three important aspects for interpreting connectivity results, as well as briefly covering some highly complementary lines of research.

Interpreting resting state functional connectivity results, particularly at a biological or mechanistic level, is extremely challenging and often contentious. Given the complexities involved, it is not currently possible to provide a simple set of guidelines that describe the "right way" to interpret your findings. Instead, this chapter aims to give you a better understanding of the key issues that you need to think about when you try to interpret and write up your own results (or when critically reading other papers). These key issues include important underlying aspects of functional connectivity that can often end up being somewhat neglected when thinking about the interpretation.

# 6.1 The impact of psychology

One of the most common criticisms of resting state fMRI research is the inherent lack of control over the cognitive processes that occur in the brain during a resting state scan. The minimal instructions and lack of external demands on the subject during a resting state scans means that it is likely that there are large variations in what the subjects are "doing" in the scanner, both between subjects, and within the same subject from one scan to the next. Research has shown that despite this inherent variability, functional connectivity networks can be found with high consistency and reliability. Nevertheless, it is important to consider the role of ongoing psychological processes when interpreting resting state findings. Note that even in the context of task fMRI, where more specific instructions and stimuli are used, it is still impossible to have full control of psychological processes.

## 6.1.1 State versus trait influences

One common aim of resting state studies is to address research questions related to individual differences, such as: "how does functional connectivity vary as a function of intelligence, or trait anxiety," etc. The underlying assumption is that people can be characterized by a set of behavioral, emotional, and personality *traits* that are stable within individuals over time. Gaining an understanding of how functional connectivity measures vary across individuals in association with these traits is an important step for the potential use of functional connectivity as a biomarker for clinical disorders (which typically lie on the extreme end of the continuous range of a trait scale).

While traits are defined as stable characteristics over time, the *state* of a subject reflects current, temporary levels of arousal and emotional affect. The subject's state is often the result of the situation and environment, and can fluctuate quickly over time. As such, the state of the subjects during the resting state scan is a potential source of large variability and should be taken into consideration when interpreting findings. In this section we will discuss a few different psychological states that are particularly likely to vary across subjects and scans in the MRI environment. Specifically, we will focus on state arousal (sleepiness) and emotional state (specifically anxiety).

Levels of *arousal* are likely to vary quite strongly across subjects, across scans, and within the course of a single scan. The reason for this is that it is not easy to stay fully awake and alert whilst lying down in the scanner doing nothing at all (despite the instructions, which typically include telling the subject to stay awake and not think about anything in particular). It has been shown that the probability of your subject being awake inside the scanner drops drastically within the first five minutes. The likelihood of subjects falling asleep is also influenced by other factors, such as: the scanning duration and conditions (more likely to fall asleep with eyes closed or in low light), the level of experience the subject has with the environment, and the emotional state of the subjects.

The effect that sleep has on functional connectivity, and on the BOLD signal more generally, varies depending on the stage of sleep (i.e., the effects are different between light, deep, and rapid eye movement sleep). Generally speaking, sleep results in a reduction in thalamo-cortical connectivity and also alters connectivity in many resting state networks including visual, dorsal attention, and default mode networks. Nevertheless, the gross structure of resting state networks has been shown to persist in states of altered consciousness such as sleep and various levels of anesthesia. It is important to consider the potential influence of differences in arousal level across subjects as well as changes within a scan. In order to be able to assess the influence of arousal during the analysis stage, it can be helpful to obtain additional measures, such as in-scanner eye-tracker data, or post-scan self-report rating data regarding sleep quality and quantity in the night before the scan, and the level of sleepiness experienced during the scan.

The emotion that is most likely to vary in the scanner environment is anxiety. In any fMRI study, it is likely that some participants are a little claustrophobic, whereas others may be entirely comfortable in confined spaces, and yet others may have participated in studies before and, therefore, have experience with the MRI environment. These different subjects are likely to enter different emotional states when put into the scanner. Additionally, the state anxiety might change over the course of the scan as subjects become accustomed to their surroundings and the scanner noises. In general, such potential within– and between–subject fluctuations in the subjects' state are particularly important to consider in research that aims to study cross-subject trait measures like trait anxiety, stress, and depression that may be closely linked to within-subject state anxiety. In such individual difference studies, the subjects' (time-varying) state could potentially dominate and, therefore, any trait-related differences in functional connectivity across subjects may be difficult to detect. In these studies, careful consideration of the study design is required. For example, it may be possible to familiarize all subjects with the MRI environment prior to the scan using a dummy fMRI setup.

## 6.1.2  State-dependent resting state fMRI

It is also possible to turn the fact that the state of the subject can vary rapidly over the course of a scan into a key aspect of your experiment. For example, an experimental manipulation can be used to induce different states (for example, to induce stress), and resting state fMRI data can be obtained before and after this manipulation. Additionally, *steady-state paradigms* can be used, in which subjects are shown continual, ongoing stimuli such as movies or continuously moving dots. These types of steady-state stimuli are different from typical task fMRI because no discrete events occur (and no interleaved task-free periods). Instead, a steady-state approach may help obtain data with higher degrees of control over the state of the subject, and this data can subsequently be analyzed in a functional connectivity framework.

Experimental paradigms that involve state manipulations or steady-state stimuli allow us to address specific research questions and test hypotheses regarding functional connectivity. Such paradigms can be considered as an alternative to pure resting state acquisitions, depending on the nature of the research question. For example, if the aim of a study is to identify changes in functional connectivity associated with anxiety, the researcher might decide to perform the experiment in three different ways: i) a pure resting state acquisition in subjects with high versus low levels of trait anxiety, or ii) acquiring data in subjects with high and low levels of trait anxiety while presenting a calming steady-state stimulus, or iii) a stress manipulation in order to create a state of anxiety in a homogeneous group of participants (with resting state measurements being taken before and after the manipulation). The advantage of the first approach is the potential for finding clinical markers, because feasible markers are preferably obtained with pure resting state as it is easier to acquire in clinical practice. The advantage of the second approach is that the steady-state stimulus may help provide an additional level of control over the emotional state and psychological processes of the subjects compared with pure resting state. Lastly, the third approach benefits from reduced problems with cross-subject variability, because the comparison between low and high anxiety is performed within the same subjects, and may also provide greater control over the subjects' state anxiety compared with pure rest. Any of these three experiments may be of interest, although the interpretation of the findings would differ between the three approaches. As such, researchers should carefully consider all of the options for data acquisition and decide on the approach that best matches their specific research interests before embarking on a functional connectivity study.

### 6.1.3 Ongoing psychological processes when the mind is at rest

In addition to a subjects' emotional and arousal state during the scan, a further psychological aspect to consider is the cognitive state of the subject. The thought-processes that are going on when the mind is at rest have been broadly classified in terms of *stimulus independent thought* (SIT) and *stimulus oriented thought* (SOT). SIT is an internally oriented state (also called *"mind wandering"* or *"mental simulation"*), which can either be future oriented (planning) or past oriented (autobiographical memory retrieval). SIT often involves many high-level cognitive processes such as mental imagery, theory of mind and even meta awareness of the mind wandering. SOT, on the other hand, is an externally oriented state of heightened vigilance for potential upcoming external stimuli, that is also called "watchfulness" or "exploratory state."

To measure the psychological thought processes that subjects are experiencing, a common approach is to use "experience sampling probes." In this method, subjects are asked questions about their subjective experience at random intervals. For example, subjects may be asked whether they are currently thinking about something that is not linked to what they are doing at this moment (i.e., a "yes" answer is evidence of SIT). These thought probes are often used during an external task (sometimes using low versus high engagement tasks), instead of during resting state. Regions from the default mode network are often of key interest in these studies.

As suggested above, SIT and SOT are two cognitive interpretations that are of particular importance in relation to the Default Mode Network (DMN). Task-based fMRI and PET studies have shown a relationship between levels of DMN activity and levels of engagement in a task, such that regions of the DMN show a decrease in neural activity when the brain is engaged in any type of external task, compared with a higher level of neural activity at rest. Therefore, the type of spontaneous cognition that occurs at rest might be of direct importance to the interpretation of the DMN. Previous findings have linked DMN activation and functional connectivity to aspects of both SIT and SOT. It is possible that these two cognitive hypotheses about the DMN are not mutually exclusive, and that the mind switches between states of internally oriented attention (SIT) and externally oriented attention (SOT). Note that the relative contribution of SIT and SOT may vary over the course of a day, so scans obtained early in the morning may differ from a psychological point of view to scans obtained later in the day.

## 6.2  The effects of BOLD physiology

As we have discussed in the previous chapters of this book, fMRI resting state functional connectivity methods aim to describe similarities between the BOLD signal timecourses obtained
from separate spatial locations in the brain. However, as explained briefly in Chapter 1, the
BOLD signal is an indirect measure of neuronal activity and reflects a complex interaction
between neural activity, blood flow, and ensuing change of the blood volume. When activity increases in a neuronal population, this results in a localized increase in blood flow and
volume. The supply of oxygenated blood to the active region exceeds the oxygen demands
of that region. Therefore, neural activity leads to an increase in the amount of oxygenated
blood in the activated brain region, which results in a positive change in the BOLD signal
measured with fMRI. From this brief description it is clear that many intermediate processes
occur between the neurons firing and the change in the local concentration of deoxygenated
hemoglobin that is measured by the BOLD signal.

A further important aspect of the BOLD signal is the cross-subject and cross-region variability
in the hemodynamic response function. Blood flow starts to increase within seconds after the
increase of neuronal activity, and only peaks approximately six seconds after the neuronal activity. This is a very longtime scale compared with that of neural firing, which typically occurs at
the rate of milliseconds. This means that the BOLD signal measured in fMRI is not only an
indirect measure, but also a delayed and temporally imprecise measure of neuronal activity.
Note that the caveats of interpreting the BOLD signal discussed in the rest of this section are
not exclusively associated with resting state functional connectivity research. In any study that
uses BOLD data, these considerations should be taken into account when interpreting results.

An important implication of its indirect nature is that the BOLD signal relates to the amount
of perturbations of the magnetic field due to the differences between oxygenated and
deoxygenated hemoglobin, and is not a direct quantitative measure. This implies that the value
of the BOLD signal cannot be interpreted in absolute terms. Hence, when we measure a BOLD
signal of 1000 from my prefrontal cortex and a BOLD signal of 2000 from your prefrontal cortex, this does not mean that there is twice as much neural activity in your prefrontal cortex than
in mine. There are many different factors that influence the BOLD values measured, ranging
from the scanner hardware and preprocessing steps, to whether or not we had a cup of coffee
before the scan and many other sources of noise. As a result of the fact that the BOLD signal is
not quantitative, we always need to analyze the data in relative terms. In the case of functional
connectivity, this is achieved by comparing the BOLD signals from two or more regions of the
same brain to each other and assessing the similarity of the ongoing signals in these regions.

### 6.2.1  Electrophysiology correlates of BOLD

Using concurrent electrophysiological and BOLD recording, it has been shown that the BOLD
signal is most strongly related to *synchronized postsynaptic activity* (which measures the summed
excitatory inputs to the neurons), and not to neural firing rates. Therefore, resting state fMRI
measurements predominantly represent fluctuations in the summed inputs to a population of
neurons, and not the output of those neurons.

For some populations of neurons, there is a direct link between the inputs and outputs, and in this case the BOLD signal is equally strongly associated with neural firing and with summed postsynaptic inputs to the neurons. However, in other regions the link between inputs to the neural region and the outputs (firing) of that region can be more complex. For example, if some neurons in the population increase their firing rate, but others decrease their firing rate (as a result of inhibitory neurons), this could lead to a net change in firing rate across the neuronal population that is close to zero. Nevertheless, an increase in BOLD signal would be measured based on the postsynaptic inputs to the neuronal population. An example of this occurs in the cerebellum, where a dissociation between firing rate and blood flow occurs as a result of inhibitory interneurons, which cause an increase in blood flow, but reduce the spiking activity of purkinje neurons.

The fact that the BOLD signal is most likely driven by the summed inputs to a population of neurons is helpful to keep in mind when looking at functional connectivity results. For example, a correlation between the BOLD signal from a cortical region and from a cerebellar region suggests a coupling between the inputs to these neuronal regions. However, in this example the neural activity of the regions (i.e., the firing rates they produce in response to the inputs) may differ strongly due to the non-linear relationship between input and output in the cerebellum.

### 6.2.2  The vascular basis of BOLD

To help us interpret changes in resting state functional connectivity, it is useful to have an understanding of how increases in excitatory input to a population of neurons lead to a localized increase in blood flow. The active process that links this postsynaptic activity to increased blood flow and volume to the region is called *neurovascular coupling*, and this process mediates the signal measured in resting state fMRI.

Given that neurovascular coupling is driving the signal that is actually measured, any changes in functional connectivity in resting state fMRI that we observe could either reflect neuronal changes in postsynaptic activity (as we would hope), or they may reflect a change in some aspect of the neurovascular coupling without any changes in neural activity. When interpreting resting state fMRI findings, it is helpful to be aware of the fact that changes in neurovascular coupling can directly affect the BOLD signal. For example, caffeine acts as a vasoconstrictor in the brain, meaning that the total amount of blood flow to your brain can reduce by as much as 20–30% after drinking a double espresso.

Neurovascular coupling is a term that describes the effects of several complex chemical processes that involve all the different types of cells that exist in a population of neurons. The hemodynamic response primarily occurs through *vasodilation*, meaning that arterioles that supply local gray matter with oxygenated blood, dilate (increase in diameter) to allow a larger volume of blood to flow into the region. While the processes giving rise to vasodilation are not yet fully understood, several chemicals are effective vasodilators and are likely to cause this increase in blood flow (including potassium and hydrogen ions). These vasoactive substances are released by processes that occur within neurons, astrocytes, and interneurons in response to increased synaptic input to the neural population. A more detailed description of the complex biochemical processes that give rise to vasodilation is beyond the scope of this primer, although further information can be found elsewhere in the literature (see Further reading).

Importantly, many of the processes that result in the release of vasoactive substances rely on the presence of intracellular calcium. This means that differences in intracellular levels of calcium between two regions, or between different subjects in a study, could have important effects on the measured BOLD signal. As such, it is possible that observed differences in functional connectivity may be driven by different levels of intracellular calcium between, for example, healthy controls and patient groups. Calcium regulation is known to be dysfunctional in a large variety of disorders including epilepsy, pathological pain, bipolar disorder, depression, schizophrenia, neurodegenerative disorders such as Alzheimer's disease and Parkinson's disease, and autoimmune diseases such as multiple sclerosis. As such, it is helpful to consider the potential role of intracellular calcium levels when interpreting functional connectivity findings, particularly in clinical populations where calcium regulation may be altered.

# 6.3 The effects of methodological choices

The breadth of preprocessing options discussed in Chapter 3, and the variety of functional connectivity measures covered in Chapters 4 and 5 can clearly give rise to a large number of different analysis pipelines for resting state fMRI data. Combined with the parameters, thresholds, and other minor decisions within each approach, the likelihood of two datasets being analyzed in exactly the same way becomes small. While this is not necessarily problematic, it does have implications for reporting and for interpretation, which are discussed below.

## 6.3.1 Guidelines for analysis and reporting

As a result of the large variety in preprocessing and analysis approaches, it is important that reporting of the methods in journal articles is detailed and comprehensive. To help optimize the transparency of analysis approaches and reporting, some guidelines have been published by the Committee on Best Practice in Data Analysis and Sharing (*COBIDAS*) of the Organization for Human Brain Mapping (OHBM). These guidelines are aimed at general fMRI reporting, and are highly relevant to resting state functional connectivity research. A short summary of the COBIDAS guidelines is discussed below, but please see the full guidelines (Further reading) for much more information.

When writing up your resting state study, it is important to clearly describe each aspect of your study, including:

- The subjects that took part (including sample details and inclusion/exclusion criteria);
- The instructions given to the subjects (for resting state this includes aspects such as eyes open, fixation);
- The acquisition parameters for the scan (field strength, voxel size, TR, TE, multiband factor, etc.);
- The preprocessing steps that were performed, including the parameters used where relevant;
- The analysis steps that were performed.

The preprocessing pipelines in functional connectivity studies are often complex and typically include many different steps. Therefore, it is essential to describe the details of each step, including the software that was used and the software version (e.g., FSL 5.0.8). Additionally, a clear description of the order in which preprocessing steps were applied to the data is important. When using in-house software, it is strongly recommended to make the code available online, to improve transparency and replicability.

When it comes to the functional connectivity analysis itself, it is important to include details of the analysis. For example, when running a group-ICA decomposition it is important to describe the data entered into the group-ICA as well as the dimensionality. When running any type of node-based analysis, provide details of how the nodes (ROIs) were defined, and describe whether full or partial correlation was used, and if any regularization of these values was applied.

In terms of the statistics used to perform a group-level analysis, make sure to describe the test statistic, the group-level test that was performed (e.g., paired $t$-test), as well as the method for estimating and thresholding the $p$-value (e.g., permutation testing). When writing up the findings, it is important to be inclusive and present all of the results from the analysis, instead of selectively reporting only some of the results based on whether they fit hypotheses, or are easily interpretable. Another important factor to report is what types of nuisance variables were included in the group GLM analysis. Examples of commonly used nuisance variables at the group-level include sex, age, intracranial volume, and subject-wise summary measures of head motion.

In summary, it is very important in resting state fMRI studies to pay careful attention to the write up of the methods that were adopted. Generally speaking, the reader should have a thorough and complete understanding of how your study was performed (and should be able to replicate the pipeline) after reading the article, so including detailed descriptions is crucial. Carefully described methods sections also ensure that other researchers are able to adopt a comparable analysis pipeline, thereby facilitating an independent replication of findings.

## 6.3.2  Visualization of functional connectivity results

In addition to writing up the methods section in a transparent and sufficiently detailed way, another important aspect that is closely related to interpretation is how to visualize the functional connectivity results in a succinct and interpretable format.

For voxel-based methods, visualization is relatively straightforward, as the result from these methods is typically a whole-brain map of statistical values. These maps can be displayed using visualization packages available in many of the most commonly used fMRI analysis software packages, including AFNI, SPM, and FSL. When using these tools, it is often necessary to change the display range and potentially to change the colors (for example to view both positive and negative results). For interpretation of results, it is sometimes useful to change the display range in order to look at results that did not pass significance thresholding. An example of this is a situation where you find a significant result in a right lateralized region, but not in the homologous left lateralized region. It may be tempting to interpret this in terms of a lateralization effect (i.e., the right region is involved and the left is not). However, it is possible that the left region showed essentially the same effect, but this effect was marginally weaker and, therefore, the right side just survived statistical thresholding and the left side did not. This would lead to a very different interpretation than that suggested above. In general, it is not possible to draw any conclusions from the lack of a significant result, because it can either mean that there was no effect, or it could mean that it was just under the threshold (as in the example above), and there was just not enough statistical power to find it. In summary, it is important to think about the image that you are viewing: what do the values represent, and which range of the test statistics is the most interesting?

Visualization of node-based methods is slightly more challenging, because we are typically interested in the edges (connections) between regions, and not in the nodes themselves. When it comes to visualizing node-based results, there are many options available and each of these options emphasize different aspects of the results (Figure 6.1). For example, in some cases it might be important to emphasize the anatomical location of the nodes, by plotting the results on top of a brain. However, given the three-dimensional nature of the brain, it can become difficult to see individual edges in this layout. Therefore, it may be preferable to use visualizations where edges are more clearly visible, such as a *connectogram*, network matrix or graph. It is still possible to include some anatomical information in these options, for example by grouping nodes together based on their functionality (e.g., grouping sensorimotor nodes together, separately from DMN nodes). A variety of different software packages are available for the visualization of node-based connectivity results.

One feature that is appearing more often in recently developed visualization packages is the ability to interactively view seed-based correlation maps. Hence, in some packages it is possible to "point and click" at any region in the brain in order to view the whole-brain seed-based connectivity map using the region you clicked on as a seed. This can be helpful for exploring the dataset and checking consistency with previous findings, but is not a replacement for more thorough functional connectivity analyses. The large set of maps that are being produced when we treat each voxel as an individual seed region and calculate the whole-brain seed-based correlation map for each voxel is known as the "*dense connectome*." Visualization of dense connectomes is a feature in the "Workbench Viewer" in "Connectome Workbench," developed as part of the Human Connectome Project (www.humanconnectome. org), and some other visualization packages.

In summary, there are many good options available for visualizing functional connectivity results. When deciding which option to use for publishing your work, it is important to consider which aspect deserves most emphasis depending on your hypothesis, methods, and findings.

### 6.3.3 Relationship between methods choice and interpretation

All of the analysis options described in Chapters 4 and 5 broadly relate to some aspect of functional connectivity. However, there are important differences in the specific way in which you would interpret the results from the different types of functional connectivity analysis methods. Hopefully the descriptions of the methods and the discussion of advantages and disadvantages that were included in Chapters 4 and 5 have helped to give you an understanding of these differences in interpretation. Here, we will first discuss a brief example to provide a direct comparison between the types of results that can be obtained from all of the different methods included in this primer (Table 6.1). After this, we show two sets of results obtained

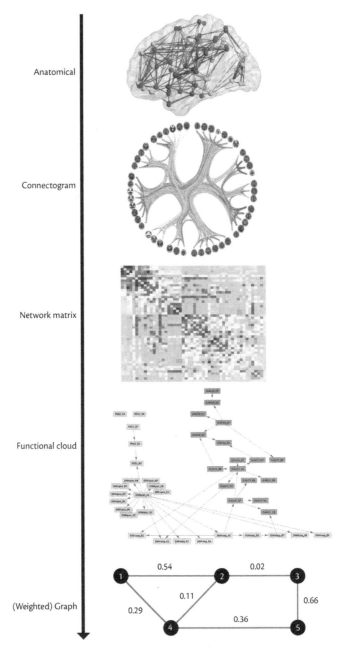

Anatomical

Connectogram

Network matrix

Functional cloud

(Weighted) Graph

**Figure 6.1:** When it comes to visualizing node-based functional connectivity results there are many options available for representing the findings. These visualization options fall on a continuum that ranges from anatomical visualization (represented on a brain), through connectograms (where the figures on the outside of the circle show the spatial location of the nodes, therefore containing some anatomical information) to matrices and graphs (more abstract representations). The best visualization option depends on the hypothesis of the study, the methods adopted, and the findings. A larger version of the connectogram figure can be found on the cover, and a more detailed version of the network matrix figure is in given in Figure 5.2.

from identical data by adopting different analysis approaches, and discuss how these two sets of results might be interpreted.

For this first example, imagine that you acquired resting state fMRI data from two different groups of subjects, namely a group of subjects who are currently suffering from Major Depression Disorder (MDD), and a group of matched subjects with no history of depression (healthy controls; HC). The aim of the study is to determine differences in functional connectivity between the MDD and HC groups. We are going to assume that different types of analysis are being performed on the data, and in each case the group-level analysis is a one-sided unpaired $t$-test for MDD lower than HC (note that this comparison is only intended as an example test that might be performed; in the absence of hypotheses on the directionality of the finding, it would be important to investigate changes in either direction). Table 6.1 contains brief descriptions of the kinds of results that you would obtain when performing the same group-level comparisons depending on the type of functional connectivity analysis method chosen. The statements in Table 6.1 do not reflect true functional connectivity findings in major depressive disorder. Instead, the aim of the table is to provide a summary of all of the measures discussed in this primer, and MDD is only used as an example so that you can begin to think about how results might be interpreted. Of course, the details included below are specific to this example, and should be changed according to the type of group comparison that is being performed.

Table 6.1 An example showing the different results that can be obtained from a functional connectivity analysis, depending on the chosen analysis method. For each method, results are from a group analysis that compares patients with depression (MDD) to healthy controls (HC) in a one-sided $t$-test (MDD<HC). The interpretation of findings can become complicated, particularly if connectivity is negative in one or both of the subject groups (as mentioned briefly in the dual regression box in the table, and discussed later in this chapter). Note that this table does not reflect findings related to MDD in the literature, instead any statements regarding MDD should be considered as examples.

| Voxel-based methods | |
| --- | --- |
| **Method** | **Result** |
| Seed-based correlation analysis | Whole-brain map showing regions of the brain with significantly lower connectivity with the seed region in MDD patients compared with HC. |
| Dual regression analysis (driven by either group ICA or other network maps) | One whole-brain map for each of the components. Taking the DMN as an example, this map identifies regions in the brain that showed significant lower connectivity with the DMN as a whole, in MDD compared with HC (including regions where connectivity with the DMN is strongly negative in MDD patients, but close to zero or positive in HC). This can include both regions that are within the DMN in the group map, or regions that are outside the DMN, but that still show a significant difference in their connectivity with the DMN between the two subject groups. In both cases, the significant voxels essentially participate less in DMN processes in the MDD group compared with HC. |

*(continued)*

**Table 6.1** Continued

| Voxel-based methods | |
| --- | --- |
| **Method** | **Result** |
| Amplitude of low frequency fluctuations | Whole-brain map showing regions of the brain with significantly reduced (fractional) low frequency power in the MDD patients compared with HC subjects. |
| Regional homogeneity | Whole-brain map showing regions of the brain that had significantly lower timeseries similarity with neighboring voxels in MDD patients compared with HC subjects. |
| **Node-based methods** | |
| **Method** | **Result** |
| Network modeling analysis | Matrix that shows which edges between pairs of nodes had significantly reduced full or partial correlation in MDD patients compared with HC subjects. |
| Graph theory analysis | Findings often include both global and local graph theoretic measures. For example, HC subjects may show increased global efficiency compared with MDD patients. Additionally, a graph may be included, which identifies which of the nodes showed a significant decrease in node centrality in MDD patients compared with HC. |
| Dynamic causal modeling | Typically involves a single group-level analysis to compare different model configurations and determine which directional model best fits all of the data, and therefore it is not common to compare two groups against each other (although there are exceptions to this; for example, DCM has been used to identify sub-groups within heterogeneous patient populations). For the group as a whole, the result would be the relative evidence across different models, as well as the configuration and weights of the best fitting model in the form of a matrix of directional edges that describe the strength, as well as the direction of each connection. This is often visualized as a graph with arrows. |

When interpreting the findings from any functional connectivity method, it is important to consider the advantages and disadvantages of the method you chose to use. For example, when looking at the results of a fractional amplitude of low frequency fluctuations analysis, it is helpful to keep in mind that this approach does not explicitly measure functional connectivity and is, therefore, relatively sensitive to non-neuronal fluctuations. In general, being aware of the strengths and weaknesses of the analysis method will allow you to interpret and discuss your findings in the most appropriate and balanced way.

As a further example of the different ways that you might interpret results from different functional connectivity methodologies (particularly between voxel-based and node-based methods), we performed two different analyses on the same dataset. We used data from the Human Connectome Project, and performed a group comparison between 100 subjects who scored the lowest on a test of fluid intelligence (done outside the scanner), and 100 subjects with the highest scores on the same test. The group comparisons were performed using either a voxel-based dual regression approach (Figure 6.2), or using a node-based network modeling analysis (Figure 6.3). Each of these results are discussed briefly below, focusing on the way these findings could be interpreted. These analyses were performed for illustrative purposes to provide a tangible example of the different approaches and related interpretations. These findings have not been published or validated, and any statements regarding fluid intelligence should be considered as examples only.

An example dual regression result (based on low-dimensional group-ICA networks) is shown in Figure 6.2. The yellow-orange regions reflect the thresholded group-level ICA component that the results are derived from (i.e., component 6 out of 25, which is the frontoparietal network; two further group-ICA components revealed significant dual regression results, but are not shown here). The areas highlighted in green are the regions in which subjects with high fluid intelligence showed stronger connectivity with this component compared to subjects

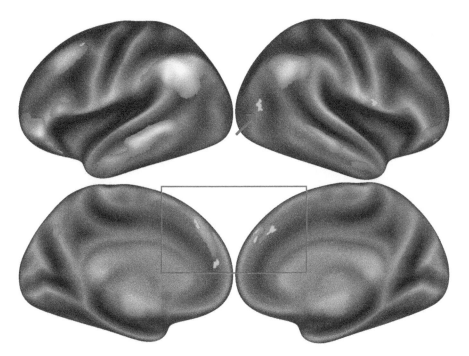

**Figure 6.2:** Example of a dual regression result from a comparison of 100 low- and 100 high-scoring subjects on a fluid intelligence task (using data from the Human Connectome Project). Areas shown in yellow–orange reflect the group-ICA component that these findings relate to, which in this case is the frontoparietal network. The results of a group comparison between high and low scoring subjects are shown in green (these results were corrected for multiple comparisons using false discovery rate thresholding). The findings show increased connectivity between the frontoparietal network and medial prefrontal regions (within the blue square), as well as the temporal–parietal–occipital junction (highlighted by the blue arrow).

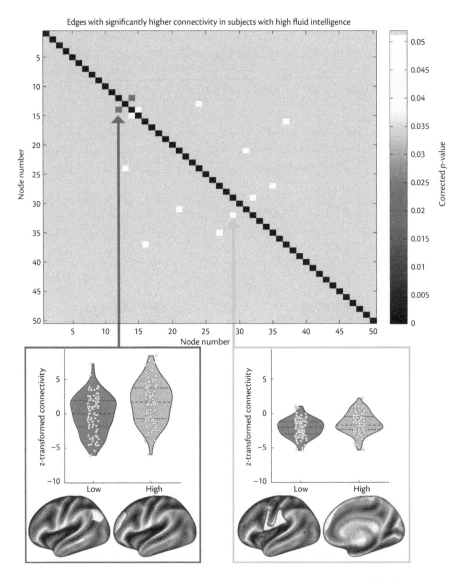

**Figure 6.3:** Example of node-based network modelling results from a comparison of 100 low- and 100 high-scoring subjects on a fluid intelligence task (using HCP data). The example findings show increased connectivity between the dorsolateral prefrontal cortex and the lateral parietal cortex that is part of the DMN, in subjects with higher fluid intelligence scores (blue box). Additionally, connectivity between the pars opercularis and the medial prefrontal cortex was more strongly negative in subjects with lower fluid intelligence scores, and closer to zero in subjects with higher scores (green box). The violin plots at the bottom show Z-transformed correlations between the two nodes.

with low fluid intelligence (i.e., the BOLD timecourses of these regions were more similar to the BOLD timecourse of the network in those who scored highly). It is clear that some green regions occur within (or on the borders of) the frontoparietal network (for example in the medial prefrontal cortex), whereas other green regions occur entirely outside of the frontoparietal network. These findings may be interpreted by saying that subjects who score highly on the fluid intelligence task showed stronger and more extensive connectivity between medial prefrontal regions and the frontoparietal network (Figure 6.2, square). Additionally, high-scoring subjects displayed connectivity between the right temporal-parietal-occipital (TPO) junction and the frontoparietal network, whereas this edge was not significantly different from zero in low-scoring subjects (Figure 6.2, arrow). The latter is of particular interest because the right TPO junction is known to be involved in spatial awareness, so increased connectivity between this region and the frontoparietal network in those who perform well on a task that requires abstract spatial processing is consistent with known function.

The same group comparison was performed on a node-based network analysis using nodes obtained from a higher dimensional ICA, and the results are displayed in Figure 6.3. Edges in which subjects with high fluid intelligence scores had significantly higher partial correlation compared with low-scoring subjects are shown on the 50–by–50 node network matrix. A total of seven edges showed a significant difference after FDR-correction for multiple comparisons, and two of these edges are visualized and discussed in more detail. First, the partial correlation between the lateral parietal node (part of the DMN network), and the bilateral dorsolateral prefrontal cortex (DLPFC) node was higher in subjects with high fluid intelligence and close to zero in subjects with lower scores. An interpretation of this might be that subjects with higher fluid intelligence scores display functional coupling between the lateral parietal node of the DMN and the DLPFC, while people with lower scores do not show this coupling. This finding was not seen in the dual regression results presented above, because the dual regression finding only involved changes in connectivity of the frontoparietal network (when looking at dual regression results in the DMN these node-based findings were also not evident, which may be due to more stringent corrections for multiple comparisons across the whole brain).

The second node-based example result involves the partial connectivity between the medial prefrontal cortex and the pars opercularis. The interpretation of this finding is more complicated due to the fact that there was strong negative connectivity (i.e., an anticorrelation) between these two nodes for subjects with lower scores on fluid intelligence, and this was reduced (i.e., closer to zero) in subjects with higher scores. Interestingly, this result involves the same medial prefrontal cortex region that was shown in the dual regression results in Figure 6.2, but emphasizes its connectivity with a different node. This finding could be interpreted by saying that negative connectivity between the medial prefrontal cortex and pars opercularis is detrimental for fluid intelligence. However, interpreting (changes in) negative connectivity is even more challenging than interpreting positive connectivity, because the biological mechanisms that are involved are even less well understood, and because different preprocessing strategies can affect the presence and strength of negative correlations.

Hopefully, this side-by-side comparison of the results that can be obtained from a typical voxel-based analysis and a typical node-based analysis provides a helpful example, and a starting point for thinking about interpreting your own findings. It is important to appreciate, however, that the interpretation of any specific set of results depends highly on the research question, the experimental setup, the methods chosen, and the aim of the study. For example, if the aim of the study is to understand the functional connectivity substrates of fluid intelligence, then the finding of increased connectivity between the TPO junction and the frontoparietal network may be sufficiently informative in its own right. However, if the aim is to identify a biomarker for fluid intelligence, then further analyses (using multivariate classification/prediction methods) would be required to determine the accuracy with which TPO-frontoparietal connectivity is able to predict fluid intelligence.

From the comparison of voxel-based and node-based results it is clear that different findings can be obtained from different methods (even though these are all functional connectivity methods). The reasons for this may be a combination of (i) inherent differences in the sensitivity of specific approaches to different findings, (ii) differences in the dimensionality of the analysis (i.e., voxel-based methods are typically used to investigate a small number of large-scale networks, whereas node-based methods often involve a larger number of spatially smaller nodes), and (iii) differences in multiple comparison correction and thresholding. As such, it is worthwhile spending some time to decide which functional connectivity method to adopt. When making this decision, you should take into account the existing literature (is there prior knowledge for which regions will be most interesting, or is this unknown?), and the research question (e.g., is the aim to identify neural connectivity substrates, or to come up with biomarkers).

## 6.3.4  Connectivity: functional, effective, or anatomical

There are three different types of connectivity that can be differentiated, which include functional connectivity (the main type of connectivity discussed in this primer), as well as effective and anatomical connectivity. To help guide the interpretation of your connectivity findings, it is helpful to have a good grasp of these different connectivity concepts.

By now you will hopefully be very familiar with functional connectivity, which describes temporal relationships between signals from spatially distinct regions of the brain. However, as you can see from this description, the concept of functional connectivity is relatively abstract because it essentially describes a statistical property of the data we measure, rather than biological processes. Of course, when we come to interpret functional connectivity results, we typically discuss findings in terms of functional integration or functional coupling. Hence, functional connectivity is thought to reflect transfer of information across connections between different neural populations. There is evidence from multimodal studies that shows that functional connectivity is grounded in biology, and this is discussed a bit more in the next section on complementary types of connectivity research. Nevertheless, it is useful to keep in mind that functional connectivity is, at its heart, a relatively abstract statistical concept.

Of the different types of connectivity, *anatomical connectivity* (also called *structural connectivity*), is the most strongly grounded in biology. Anatomical connectivity simply refers to the presence or absence of white matter tracts between neural populations (i.e., the presence of "wiring" between regions). Anatomical connectivity plays an important role in mapping the connectome, and can be investigated using diffusion MRI or tract tracing (in animals).

It is worth highlighting at this stage that it is possible to find evidence of functional connectivity, even when there is no direct anatomical connection between two regions. This does not necessarily mean that the functional connectivity finding is wrong, because the brain is essentially one highly connected system. The way this type of finding is often interpreted is to say that the two regions are *indirectly* connected. Hence, in this scenario the most likely reason for the functional connectivity finding is that both regions have anatomical and functional connections to a third region (or to a complex set of regions), such that information is passed between the two regions via this third region (i.e., indirectly). As described in Chapter 5, partial correlation is a node-based method that is less sensitive to such indirect connections. A further possibility is that a true anatomical connection does exist, but is not measured in diffusion MRI. This can, for example, occur in cases where the white matter fibers are not myelinated (or are very thin), or when there is a complex configuration of fibers.

Once you know about the functional as well as the anatomical connectivity between two regions, there is still one question unanswered, namely: what is the direction of the information flow for any particular connection? *Effective connectivity* is defined as the degree of direct influence that one neural population exerts on another neural population. Similarly to functional connectivity (although to a lesser extent), effective connectivity is a relatively abstract term. Biologically speaking, it is likely that many connections between different brain regions are bi-directional, suggesting that both bottom-up and top-down interactions between the regions are possible. The presence of both excitatory and inhibitory connections at a neuronal level further complicates the relationship between estimated effective connectivity and the underlying neurophysiological mechanisms. Nevertheless, determining the dominant *directionality* of the information flow is of interest in terms of gaining an understanding of the connectome.

Studying effective connectivity using functional MRI data is relatively challenging. The reason for this is that many effective connectivity methods are so called lag-based methods, such as Granger causality. As we briefly discussed in Chapter 5, lag-based methods work on the assumption that if something happens first in region A and later in time in region B, then the directionality of the connection must go from region A to region B. However, due to fMRI being an indirect and sluggish measure of neuronal activity, especially relative to the time scale of neuronal events (typically milliseconds), the temporal information in fMRI is limited and performing such lag-based analyses is problematic. However, lag-based methods can be successfully used in other modalities, as discussed briefly in the next section. Alternatively, other methods that do not rely on temporal lag may be able to determine directionality from fMRI data.

In summary, this section discussed the three different types of connectivity, as well as closely linked topics such as indirect and directional connectivity, in a little bit more detail. When it comes to interpreting your findings, it will be helpful for those who will read your work if you use nomenclature in line with these definitions, and to keep in mind that functional connectivity is, in essence, a relatively abstract concept that is somewhat removed from the underlying neurophysiology.

## 6.4  Complementary types of connectivity research

Up until now, this primer has focused exclusively on functional connectivity analyses performed on resting state data obtained with functional MRI. The reason for this is that MRI is a non-invasive method that acquires data with relatively high spatial resolution, compared with alternative approaches. As a result, it is the most commonly used modality for functional connectivity research. Nevertheless, there are many complementary research modalities that are crucial in order to obtain a complete understanding of functional connectivity. Specifically, multi-modal approaches play a vital role to help us gain insights into the relationship between functional and anatomical connectivity, to better understand certain characteristics of connectivity (such as dynamic changes over time), and study the neurophysiological mechanisms that mediate the BOLD signal.

In this section, we discuss several important complementary approaches to studying connectivity. The aim of this section is to provide an overview of the strengths and weaknesses of these modalities, and to highlight how they can provide insights that cannot be achieved with functional MRI alone. This section is not attempting to review all of the research performed in these modalities to date. Rather, the aim is to provide insights into how these modalities can be used to help progress our understanding of functional connectivity. If you would like to read a more general review of these fields, several review articles are highlighted in the section on Further reading.

## 6.4.1  Diffusion imaging

Perhaps the most obvious candidate for multimodal connectivity research is to look at diffusion MRI. Diffusion MRI is a non-invasive MRI approach that is sensitive to the diffusion of water molecules. Diffusion describes how the molecules spread out, like when you put a droplet of ink into a glass of water, the ink will slowly spread out from the initial drop to the whole glass. When water can move around freely, the diffusion is equal in all directions (which is called isotropic diffusion), but when there are some restrictions in the way (such as tissue boundaries), diffusion will not be equal in all directions (*anisotropic diffusion*). In white matter tracts in the brain, water diffuses more freely along the axons than perpendicular to their direction, which makes the signal sensitive to the direction of the axons and their microstructure (e.g., size, density, myelination, etc.). Common parameters that can be estimated from diffusion MRI include *mean diffusivity* (total amount of diffusion in a voxel), and *fractional anisotropy* (how anisotropic the diffusion is in a voxel). Diffusion MRI data can also be used for *tractography*, i.e., mapping entire white matter tracts in the brain. As such, diffusion MRI provides a valuable measure of anatomical connectivity that can be used non-invasively in humans.

The main strength of diffusion MRI as a complementary approach to resting state fMRI is that it allows us to determine whether or not measures of functional connectivity are related to the presence of direct anatomical connectivity. On the other hand, relative weaknesses of diffusion imaging include uncertainty about the precise location of the origin and termination of white matter tracts, being less sensitive to white matter tracts that are not myelinated, and difficulties separating complex fiber structures (such as areas containing crossing and kissing fibers). It is also important to remember that while functional connectivity can reflect both polysynaptic and mono-synaptic (indirect and direct) connectivity, diffusion MRI is only sensitive to the latter. Some of these weaknesses can be addressed by other complementary techniques discussed below, while others require post-mortem dissection to be better understood. Despite these drawbacks, diffusion MRI is a useful technique and is commonly acquired alongside resting state fMRI.

Combined diffusion MRI—resting state fMRI research has shown repeatedly that functional connectivity estimated from resting state fMRI reflects the underlying white matter structural connectivity. Therefore, diffusion MRI plays an important role in connectomics, because validation using anatomical connectivity is an important aspect of mapping out the connections in the human brain. A further advantage of acquiring both of these modalities in one study is that it can help identify any anatomical abnormality that might underlie differences in functional connectivity between patients and healthy controls. For these reasons, many resting state fMRI studies, including large-scale studies such as the Human Connectome Project, acquire diffusion MRI data in addition to resting state data for multimodal analysis and validation.

## 6.4.2 Electrophysiological methods

Electrophysiological methods such as electroencephalography (EEG) and magnetoencephalography (MEG) form another group of approaches that can help our understanding of functional connectivity in a way that cannot be achieved with resting state fMRI alone. When a neuron is active, an action potential is generated by rapidly changing the *electrical membrane potential* of a cell. This electrical activity can be measured from outside the head, either by measuring electric currents with electrodes placed on the scalp (EEG), or by measuring the magnetic fields resulting from these currents using an MEG scanner. In this section, we focus on electrophysiological measures obtained non-invasively from humans, while electrophysiology in animals is discussed further in the next section.

There are two important benefits of electrophysiological measures compared with functional MRI. First, the measurements obtained in EEG and MEG are a more direct measure of neuronal activity than fMRI, because they are not mediated by the hemodynamic response function. The second advantage is that electrophysiological measures benefit from a much better temporal resolution compared with fMRI, as they are able to obtain many measurements every second. For example, the sampling rate in EEG is typically between 200–1000 data points per second, compared with a TR of one to three seconds in fMRI (i.e., often less than one data point per second). In addition, fMRI and EEG (but not MEG) data can be acquired simultaneously, which provides a valuable opportunity for directly comparing electrophysiological and BOLD resting state measurements.

Given the high temporal resolution of EEG and MEG, a good reason for adopting these approaches is to study the temporal dynamics of functional connectivity. For example, transient brain states lasting for 200–300 milliseconds were identified using MEG. As discussed in Chapter 5, studying these fast dynamic changes in connectivity over time using fMRI is challenging because of the delay resulting from the hemodynamic response function, and electrophysiological measures, therefore, provide an important complementary technique to investigate functional connectivity at faster temporal scales.

However, an important limitation of both EEG and MEG is that it is challenging to determine the location of the activity (i.e., the source)—a challenge known as solving the *"inverse problem."* Therefore, the spatial resolution of these electrophysiological methods is poor in comparison to fMRI; at best in the region of 10 millimeters, relative to 1–3 millimeters in fMRI. Nevertheless, the far superior temporal resolution of these methods means that much can be gained from studying functional connectivity using electrophysiological approaches in conjunction with fMRI research.

Note that an invasive method called electrocorticography (ECoG) is also increasingly used to study functional connectivity in humans who require ECoG for medical reasons (e.g., for patients with epilepsy). ECoG involves placing a grid of electrodes directly on the cortical surface after removing the skull. As with MEG and EEG, the primary advantage of EGoC is the improved temporal resolution, and ECoG has, therefore, also been used to investigate the temporal and frequency characteristics of local resting state functional connectivity within the area covered by the electrodes.

### 6.4.3  Functional connectivity research in animals

The previous section focused primarily on non-invasive electrophysiological methods in humans. However, using fMRI and neural recording methods in animals has also been invaluable for our understanding of resting state fMRI data, and of the BOLD signal more generally (which was discussed in Chapter 1 and earlier in this chapter, and will not be repeated here).

The advantages of performing functional connectivity research in animals are that it allows us to perform interventional approaches (including optogenetic or electrical manipulation or pharmacological intervention), and that it enables us to study disease mechanisms using, for example, rodent models of disease. Additionally, a much wider variety of invasive neuroscientific methods can be adopted in animal research, compared with human studies. The use of a wider variety of data acquisition methods means that studies can benefit from the advantages of any particular method chosen (which often include advantages such as good signal to noise ratios, and good spatial as well as temporal resolution). For example, a mouse model was used to show a causal relationship between a deficit in microglia, and resulting autism-like impairments in social behavior, as well as resulting abnormalities in functional connectivity. This example made the most of the advantages listed above, as it used a rodent model of disease, and recorded both local field potentials in freely behaving animals as well as fMRI under anesthesia, to understand the relationship between cellular changes at the level of synapses and resulting deficits in behavior and connectivity.

One disadvantage of the use of animals to study functional connectivity (in addition to ethical reservations), is that obtaining data from animals typically involves the use of *anesthetics*. These anesthetics have been shown to reduce functional connectivity, and also induce hypercapnia (elevated levels of $CO_2$ in the blood), which affects the BOLD signal. Although studies have shown evidence of good agreement in functional connectivity networks observed in awake and anesthetized animals, the influence of anesthetics is an important disadvantage. As a result, the use of anesthetics is increasingly avoided altogether by performing awake scanning, or using advanced methods for data acquisition that can be adopted in awake and freely behaving animals.

### 6.4.4  Theoretical neuroscience and simulated neural networks

From resting state fMRI studies we know that the brain is intrinsically organized into large scale functional networks of highly connected brain regions. However, this does not provide us with a mechanistic understanding of these networks. Hence, we do not currently have a clear understanding of why the networks are structured in this way, or of what types of information processing occurs in different areas of these networks. Theoretical neuroscience aims to address these types of mechanistic questions by trying to recreate the networks that we see using simulated computational models of neural networks. Theoretical neuroscience methods work by developing biologically informed models of neural populations, and comparing the resulting organization and dynamics that emerge in these simulated models to measured data from fMRI and other modalities. The aim of theoretical neuroscience is to determine which biologically informed features are essential in order to recreate realistic functional networks.

The main advantages of simulation methods are that they can be used to establish links between different types of connectivity (e.g., structural and functional), and across multiple scales of investigation ranging from neural firing in individual neurons to larger populations and whole brain networks. Simulated neural network models have been used to show that anatomical connections are essential for the emergence of functional connectivity networks, and that functional connectivity matches anatomical connectivity across longer time scales (although variability occurs at shorter intervals). Furthermore, simulation approaches have been used to reveal that aspects such as coupling strength, conduction velocity and "noise" are essential to recreate the type of dynamic network structure that we see in the brain.

An important limitation of this approach lies in the complexity of the human brain, meaning that it is not yet feasible or interpretable to model the entire brain as a set of billions of individual neurons. A further limitation is that simulated models of neural networks necessarily involve many assumptions and simplifications (partly as a result of the first limitation of complexity), and therefore, it is important to carefully validate the findings against a wide range of measurements obtained from animal and human research using a variety of imaging modalities.

## 6.4.5  Transcranial stimulation methods

Transcranial stimulation methods use either electric signals or magnetic fields to alter the neuronal activity in a spatially localized part of the underlying brain tissue. Hence, the methods discussed in this section are not imaging methods that record data from the brain, but interventional methods that allow researchers to introduce temporary changes in neural activity. For example, transcranial direct current stimulation (tDCS) involves placing two electrodes on the scalp and passing a very low current through these electrodes. The effect of tDCS is to cause the resting membrane potential of neurons to *hyperpolarize* or *depolarize* for a short period of time. There are two types of stimulation possible with tDCS; anodal stimulation leads to increased *neuronal excitability* through cell depolarization, whereas cathodal stimulation decreases the neuronal excitability through hyperpolarization. Transcranial magnetic stimulation (TMS), an alternative stimulation method, creates a localized alternating magnetic field that induces currents in the neural tissue. TMS can, therefore, be used to directly trigger action potentials or, alternatively, patterns of TMS stimulation (such as *theta burst stimulation*) can be used to alter the neuronal excitability, in a similar way to tDCS. Both theta burst TMS and tDCS can be used to trigger temporary changes in neural firing in a relatively localized region of the brain that last for some period of time after stimulation.

The main advantage of using stimulation methods together with fMRI is that they can be used to implement experimentally controlled manipulations of local neural firing in a way that is temporary and safe to use in humans. As such, using methods such as TMS and tDCS allows us to study the causal relationships between localized neural firing and whole brain functional connectivity by means of directly manipulating a hypothesized causal connection, thereby confirming the relevance of the area. This is important to help improve our understanding of functional connectivity, as we can disrupt connectivity in a controlled manner and study the spatial and temporal results of the disruption. Methods such as TMS and tDCS may also be used as treatment approaches for disorders in which altered functional connectivity is thought to play a major role (such as depression and schizophrenia). The combined use of stimulation methods and fMRI may help shed light on dysfunctional pathways in those disorders.

An important disadvantage of transcranial stimulation methods are that there is a large amount of variability in the effects of these methods from one person to the next and from day to day. This is largely related to the fact that very small variations in the positioning of stimulation can result in large changes in the effect of the stimulation. Due to these disadvantages it is important to gain a better understanding of the physiological mechanisms that are involved in these stimulation methods, and to optimize the application of TMS and tDCS, and a lot of research is being done in these important areas. Nevertheless, stimulation methods are currently one of the very few ways in which we are able to perform interventions in healthy human subjects at the neuronal level, and therefore, these techniques play an important role in many types of neuroimaging research, including functional connectivity research.

## 6.5 Conclusions

In this final chapter of this primer, we have highlighted key aspects that should be taken into consideration when interpreting resting state functional connectivity results. Interpreting findings is challenging, and it is not uncommon to find differences of opinion between researchers as to how certain results should be described and interpreted. This potential for lack of consensus arises from the fact that the biological and physiological mechanisms that give rise to the changes in fMRI connectivity are poorly understood. Therefore, it is important to discuss your findings extensively with coauthors and collaborators, and to consider all of the factors that are important for interpretation, as described in this chapter.

This chapter also contains a summary of different types of complementary techniques, including electrophysiological, theoretical, and transcranial stimulation methods. These were specifically included in light of our lack of understanding of underlying biological mechanisms, because multimodal studies that combine different types of complementary acquisition methods are essential for investigating the link between BOLD connectivity and underlying biological processes.

After reading this primer, it should be clear that resting state functional connectivity is a research field that is still at a relatively early stage, and that it is evolving rapidly, and will most likely continue to do so over the coming years. New and improved preprocessing and analysis methods for functional connectivity are constantly being developed, and careful comparisons will become increasingly important in order to work towards a consensus on the best options for processing pipelines. Future multimodal research, that uses multiple complementary techniques, is needed to better characterize functional connectivity findings in terms of the underlying biological and physiological processes.

Functional connectivity is an exciting field to enter at this time because it is developing rapidly and is experiencing a drastic increase in the number of scientists, with a wide variety of different backgrounds and associated skillsets, contributing to the body of research. We hope that reading this primer has been useful as a starting point to enter this exciting and rapidly evolving field of neuroscience!

## SUMMARY

■ Interpretation of functional connectivity findings is an important and challenging aspect of this field of research that is complicated further by the fact that we lack a full understanding of the biological mechanisms that underlie observed changes in BOLD-derived functional connectivity.

■ When interpreting the findings, there are several things that are important to keep in mind:
  ▫ The mental state of the subject (tiredness, anxiety, and ongoing thought processes) may influence the measurement.
  ▫ BOLD data is an indirect and temporally slow measure of neuronal connectivity mediated by vasodilation.
  ▫ The interpretation of the findings should take into account the method that was used for analysis.

■ Functional connectivity research can be performed using a variety of different techniques (other than fMRI), and many of these modalities are highly complementary and essential for fully understanding the connectome.
  ▫ Diffusion imaging can be used to map structural connectivity.
  ▫ Electrophysiological measures benefit from much better temporal resolution compared with fMRI.
  ▫ Research using animal models can help progress our understanding of biological mechanisms of connectivity in healthy and disease states, because it allows for a wider range of data acquisition modalities and (pharmacological) interventions.
  ▫ Computational modeling methods can be used to simulate neural networks to gain an understanding of which features are essential for the networks we see in real data to exist.
  ▫ Transcranial stimulation methods are intervention methods that can be used to temporarily modify functional connectivity in humans.

## FURTHER READING

■ Christoff, K., Irving, Z.C., Fox, KC.R., Spreng, R.N., & Andrews-Hanna, J.R. (2016). Mind-wandering as spontaneous thought: a dynamic framework. *Nature Reviews: Neuroscience*, *17*, 718–731. Available at: http://doi.org/10.1038/nrn.2016.113.
  ▫ Review paper discussing the relationship between the DMN and spontaneous cognition.

■ Damoiseaux, J.S., & Greicius, M.D. (2009). Greater than the sum of its parts: a review of studies combining structural connectivity and resting-state functional connectivity. *Brain Structure & Function*, *213*(6), 525–533. Available at: https://doi.org/10.1007/s00429-009-0208-6.
  ▫ Literature review of multi-modal DTI–fMRI connectivity findings.

■ Deco, G., Jirsa, V.K., & McIntosh, A.R. (2013). Resting brains never rest: computational insights into potential cognitive architectures. *Trends in Neurosciences*, *36*(5), 268–274. Available at: https://doi.org/10.1016/j.tins.2013.03.001.
  ▫ Review article of theoretical neuroscience approaches.

■ Deco, G., Jirsa, V.K., & McIntosh, A.R. (2011). Emerging concepts for the dynamical organization of resting-state activity in the brain. *Nature Reviews: Neuroscience, 12*(1), 43–56. Available at: https://doi.org/10.1038/nrn2961.
    ▩ Another review article of theoretical neuroscience, that summarizes some of the key findings using simulated neural network modeling methods.

■ Gozzi, A., & Schwarz, A.J. (2016). Large-scale functional connectivity networks in the rodent brain. *NeuroImage, 127,* 496–509. Available at: http://doi.org/10.1016/j.neuroimage.2015.12.017.
    ▩ Article reviewing rodent research into large scale functional connectivity networks.

■ Lauritzen, M. (2005). Reading vascular changes in brain imaging: is dendritic calcium the key? *Nature Reviews. Neuroscience, 6*(1), 77–85. Available at: http://doi.org/10.1038/nrn1589.
    ▩ A review of the neurophysiological changes related to the BOLD signal.

■ Logothetis, N.K. (2008). What we can do and what we cannot do with fMRI. *Nature, 453*(7197), 869–878. Available at: http://doi.org/10.1038/nature06976.
    ▩ A further review of the neurophysiology that gives rise to the BOLD signal.

■ Margulies, D.S., Béttger, J., Watanabe, A., & Gorgolewski, K.J. (2013). Visualizing the human connectome. *NeuroImage, 80*(0), 445–461. Available at: https://doi.org/10.1016/j.neuroimage.2013.04.111.
    ▩ Discussion of challenges in visualizing connectivity results; contains some useful summary figures and tables with options available for visualization.

■ Nichols, T.E., Das, S., Eickhoff, S.B., Evans, A.C., Hanke, T.G.M., Kriegeskorte, N., et al. (2015). *Best Practices in Data Analysis and Sharing in Neuroimaging using MRI.* Available at: https://doi.org/10.1101/054262.
    ▩ The COBIDAS report on best practice in neuroimaging reporting. There is a specific section on connectivity analyses (5.6); however, also make sure to take a look at the checklist tables in appendix D as they contain a very helpful summary of the types of information that should be included when writing up your results.

■ Picchioni, D., Duyn, J.H., & Horovitz, S.G. (2013). Sleep and the functional connectome. *NeuroImage, 80,* 387–396. Available at: https://doi.org/10.1016/j.neuroimage.2013.05.067.
    ▩ A review of the effects of sleep on functional connectivity and many other measures.

■ Sui, J., Huster, R., Yu, Q., Segall, J.M., & Calhoun, V.D. (2014). Function-structure associations of the brain: evidence from multimodal connectivity and covariance studies. *NeuroImage, 102 Pt 1,* 11–23. Available at: https://doi.org/10.1016/j.neuroimage.2013.09.044.
    ▩ Review paper that discusses many studies that have used multiple different imaging modalities to study connectivity.

■ Zhan, Y., Paolicelli, R.C., Sforazzini, F., Weinhard, L., Bolasco, G., Pagani, F., et al. (2014). Deficient neuron-microglia signaling results in impaired functional brain connectivity and social behavior. *Nature Neuroscience, 17*(3), 400–406. Available at: https://doi.org/10.1038/nn.3641.
    ▩ Rodent study that investigates a mouse model of autism discussed in the text above.

# Index